HEALTH CO-DESIGN for COMMUNITY WELL-BEING

HEALTH CO-DESIGN for COMMUNITY WELL-BEING

VIJAYARAGHAVAN M CHARIAR
&
JAMES OLIVER

ZORBA BOOKS

ZORBA BOOKS

Published by Zorba Books, March 2026
Website: www.zorbabooks.com
Email: info@zorbabooks.com

Title: **Health Co-Design for Community Well-being**
Author Name: Vijayaraghavan M Chariar & James Oliver

Softcover ISBN :- 978-93-5896-839-2
Ebook ISBN :- 978-93-5896-941-2

Zorba Books Pvt. Ltd. (opc)
Sushant Arcade,
Next to Courtyard Marriot,
Sushant Lok 1, Gurgaon – 122009, India

Printed in India

Contents

Acknowledgements

This monograph is the collective outcome of a two-year sponsored project supported under the SPARC initiative of the Ministry of Education, Government of India. We gratefully acknowledge the Ministry's vision in supporting interdisciplinary and internationally engaged research that transcends conventional academic boundaries and enables meaningful societal engagement.

The SPARC programme provided not only financial assistance but also intellectual legitimacy for exploring health beyond disciplinary silos. By enabling collaboration among scholars, practitioners, and community knowledge holders, the initiative made it possible to nurture a dialogue that may otherwise have remained fragmented.

We extend our sincere appreciation to all contributing authors in this volume. Each chapter reflects years—often several decades—of dedicated practice across diverse health traditions and community contexts. Their willingness to articulate lived experiences, document clinical reflections, and engage in interdisciplinary dialogue has enriched this work immeasurably. This volume stands as a testament to their commitment to community well-being.

Our gratitude extends to the practitioners, patients, community members, and field collaborators whose lived realities shaped the insights presented herein. Health co-design is meaningful only when grounded in authentic engagement. The stories, challenges, and aspirations of communities provided the moral compass for this project.

We acknowledge the doctoral scholars of Frugal Innovation JoyLab., CRDT, IIT Delhi, coordinators, and administrative teams, who supported the SPARC course on "Design as Situational and Relational: Connecting to People and Place", SPARC Symposium on Health Co-Design, field visits, documentation processes, communications, and logistics throughout the project's lifecycle. Their behind-the-scenes dedication ensured continuity and rigour in execution. In particular, we are deeply indebted to SWRC, Tilonia, and Samanvaya Social Ventures for assistance with field work in Rajasthan and Auroville, respectively.

We are also thankful to institutional colleagues (at IIT Delhi and RMIT Melbourne) and peer reviewers who offered constructive critique and intellectual companionship during the development of this manuscript. Interdisciplinary work demands openness and patience, and their engagement strengthened the clarity and coherence of this volume.

Finally, we express appreciation to our families and close collaborators for their encouragement and understanding throughout the demanding phases of research, dialogue, and writing. Long-term projects are sustained not only by formal structures but also by invisible networks of emotional and moral support.

Foreword

The idea of *Health Co-Design* emerges at a time when health systems across the world are under deep reflection. The last decade has exposed structural inequities, rising chronic disease burdens, mental health crises, ecological instability, and widening trust gaps between institutions and communities. The COVID-19 pandemic further revealed the fragility of centralised models of care and the urgent need for participatory, context-sensitive approaches to well-being. It is within this moment of transition that *Health Co-Design for Community Well-being* has taken shape.

This monograph is the outcome of a two-year sponsored project under the SPARC initiative of the Ministry of Education, Government of India. The project sought not merely to examine health systems from an academic distance, but to bring together practitioners, scholars, community leaders, and traditional knowledge holders in a shared inquiry: How might we reimagine health systems if communities were not passive recipients, but equal partners in design?

Health co-design is more than a method. It is a philosophical shift. It challenges the long-standing assumption that expertise flows in one direction—from institution to community, from laboratory to field, from policy to practice. Instead, co-design positions communities as co-creators of knowledge and co-authors of solutions. It invites humility in experts and agency in citizens. It recognises that lived experience is a form of intelligence. India offers fertile ground for such a reimagination. Across its villages, towns, and cities, there exists a rich, living heritage of health practices—Ayurveda, Yoga, Siddha, Unani, Homeopathy, folk traditions, seasonal food cultures, ritual ecologies, and embodied arts. These traditions are not merely therapeutic systems; they serve as civilisational frameworks for living in harmony with the body, mind, society, and nature. Yet, despite this plurality, contemporary health discourse often remains siloed—divided by discipline, institution, and epistemology.

This volume attempts to bridge these divides. The chapters that follow reflect diverse, yet converging, pathways toward community well-being. They include practitioner accounts of Ayurvedic responses to pandemics, explorations of homeopathy as personalised care, reflections on self-care traditions within households, systems-based frameworks for participatory innovation, and artistic mediums such as music and dance as vehicles of healing. They interrogate health policies, ethical relations, plural knowledge systems, and community-led preventive care. Together, they illuminate the many dimensions of health that lie beyond hospital walls. Importantly, this monograph does not argue for the replacement of one system by another. Rather, it proposes dialogue instead of hierarchy, complementarity instead of competition, and co-learning instead of epistemic exclusion. It asks whether our health futures might be strengthened by weaving together biomedical science, traditional knowledge, community practice, and design thinking into a shared fabric of care.

The project underlying this volume was rooted in experiential engagement. Workshops, practitioner dialogues, case reflections, and interdisciplinary exchanges informed the writing of this monograph. The intent was not to produce a single authoritative narrative but to curate a chorus of voices—each grounded in lived practice, each reflective of real-world constraints and possibilities.

A central insight emerging from this collaborative journey is that sustainable health transformation cannot be engineered solely through top-down policy reform or technological innovation but must be cultivated through trust, relationship, and distributed leadership. It must honour seasonal rhythms, ecological interdependence, and social cohesion. It must create space for youth and elders alike to participate in defining what well-being means in their own contexts. Health co-design, therefore, is both pragmatic and aspirational. It is pragmatic because it addresses pressing challenges, such as non-communicable diseases, mental health stress, access inequities, and post-pandemic recovery, through participatory models that improve adoption and sustainability. It is aspirational because it imagines a future where health is not delivered but co-created; where prevention is embedded in daily life; where community intelligence shapes policy; and where dignity and agency are restored to the heart of healthcare.

This monograph is offered not as a definitive blueprint but as an invitation – to scholars, practitioners, policymakers, and community members. It invites continued experimentation, rigorous research, critical reflection, and collaborative action. It calls for evidence generation that respects plural epistemologies. It encourages educational institutions to serve as bridges rather than silos. It urges policymakers to recognise the immense human capital embedded within traditional and community-based health systems. Above all, it affirms a simple yet powerful proposition: every community holds within it the knowledge necessary to enhance its own well-being. The task before us is to create enabling architectures where this knowledge can surface, connect, evolve, and flourish.

Vijayaraghavan M. Chariar
Project Lead, SPARC Project on Health Co-Design
IIT Delhi

James Oliver
Project Co-Lead, SPARC Project on Health Co-Design
RMIT Melbourne

Perspective 1

Health Co-Design for Community Well-Being: Some Reflections

Vijayaraghavan M. Chariar
IIT Delhi

Introduction

Health co-design is emerging as a transformative and human-centred approach to shaping health and well-being solutions through meaningful involvement of communities, practitioners, researchers, and diverse knowledge holders as equal partners. At its core, health co-design recognises that the people living within a health system—individuals, families, caregivers, and community practitioners—hold insights that are essential to reimagining how health challenges are understood and addressed. Instead of viewing communities solely as beneficiaries or end users of externally designed interventions, co-design positions them as co-creators of solutions that reflect lived experiences, contextual realities, cultural values, and local intelligence.

In the context of rural India and other societies with deep civilisational histories, health co-design finds particularly fertile ground. Rural communities across India possess rich traditions of self-care, traditional medicine, seasonal health practices, food-based healing, yoga, and holistic well-being rooted in centuries of observation and close engagement with nature. Indigenous health knowledge—whether expressed through Ayurveda, Siddha, Yoga, Unani, folk healing traditions, or everyday home-based practices—has long supported preventive and promotive health. These knowledge systems are not merely medical technologies; they serve as cultural, ecological, spiritual, and relational frameworks for living well.

However, despite this extensive body of knowledge and pluralistic heritage, significant challenges persist in achieving equitable health outcomes in rural settings. Non-communicable diseases such as diabetes, hypertension, and cardiovascular disorders are increasing sharply. Mental health stressors linked to social and economic change are becoming more evident. Access to quality healthcare remains uneven, and community capacity to navigate complex health systems is often strained. One might ask: If traditional knowledge systems are so rich, why do health disparities persist? This opening paper attempts to reflect on this paradox and suggest pathways grounded in collaborative knowledge creation and participatory design.

The Promise and Philosophy of Health Co-Design

To strengthen the academic basis of this argument, it is useful to briefly trace the evolution of co-design and its relevance within health systems transformation. Originating from participatory design movements in Scandinavia during the 1970s, co-design emerged from democratic ideals that positioned workers as equal collaborators in shaping technologies that affected their lives. Over time, the principles of co-design evolved beyond industrial design into areas such as public sector innovation, education, social development, and eventually health systems.

In the health context, co-design has been reinforced by research traditions such as participatory action research, person-centred care, implementation science, and human-centred design. Across these disciplines, several shared principles recur:

- Knowledge is socially constructed and context-dependent.
- People are experts in their own lives and should guide decision-making.
- Complex challenges require iterative experimentation rather than linear solutions.
- Collaboration across differences fosters creativity, resilience, and collective insight.

Globally, co-design has been used to reshape maternal health services, mental health interventions, elder care, disability support models, and youth well-being programmes. A common insight is that when people are involved in shaping health solutions, they are more likely to adopt, sustain, and champion them. In this sense, co-design is not merely a technique—it represents a shift in power and imagination. Health co-design is rooted in the understanding that sustainable health transformation requires listening deeply to multiple voices and bridging silos across disciplines. It challenges the assumption that expert-driven systems alone can solve complex health issues. Instead, co-design promotes:

- Shared problem definition, where communities articulate their needs, aspirations, and lived challenges.
- Mutual respect among diverse knowledge traditions, acknowledging that expertise exists both inside and outside formal institutions.
- Iterative experimentation and learning, enabling adaptive and context-sensitive solutions.
- Inclusive participation, where those most affected by health issues are actively involved in shaping responses.

Co-design encourages humility. It asks health systems and practitioners to recognise what they do not yet know and to learn alongside communities rather than for them. In doing so, it offers a framework for rebalancing power, restoring dignity, and enabling community agency.

Rural Health Traditions: A Foundation for Co-Design

Rural communities in India are not passive recipients of health interventions but have historically been active stewards of their own well-being. Practices related to seasonal living, food combinations, daily routines (*dinacharya*), and menstrual health carry accumulated wisdom from generations. Local ecosystems shaped healing: forests provided medicinal plants, rivers provided therapeutic minerals, cattle contributed through milk-based preparations, and cultural rituals reinforced psychosocial resilience.

Traditional knowledge systems were integrative rather than fragmented. Health was understood as a balance—between the body and mind, individual and community, human beings and nature. The goal was not merely the absence of disease but the cultivation of vitality and purpose.

Epistemological Tensions and the Challenge of Knowledge Integration

To understand why health challenges persist despite rich cultural wisdom, we must examine the deeper epistemological tensions that shape health discourse. Traditional and modern health systems often operate from different assumptions about the body, illness, and evidence. Biomedical frameworks emphasise measurable physiological parameters and prioritise standardised interventions, while traditional frameworks prioritise balance, context, constitution, and experiential knowledge.

This divergence generates misunderstanding and mistrust. Traditional knowledge is frequently dismissed as unscientific, whereas biomedical knowledge may be perceived as impersonal and disconnected from everyday life. The question of what counts as evidence becomes a source of conflict. Community practices, despite strong experiential validation, often struggle to be accepted in policy and institutional research spaces because they do not conform to conventional scientific methodologies.

Additionally, intellectual hierarchies and institutional power structures favour top-down knowledge creation. Communities become subjects of study rather than co-authors of knowledge. Without mechanisms for co-validation and co-production of knowledge, integration remains superficial rather than transformative.

Structural Barriers to Community Well-Being

- Persistent health challenges are not only biomedical but also systemic. Among the structural issues that constrain health outcomes are:
- Fragmented care ecosystems where services, practitioners, and institutions operate in silos.
- Limited accessible health infrastructure in rural and remote regions.
- Economic precarity and migration, which disrupt

stability and intergenerational knowledge transfer.

- Urban-oriented health messaging culturally misaligned with rural realities.
- Commercial pressures that replace locally produced foods and medicines with industrial substitutes.
- Policy frameworks that focus on treatment procurement rather than community capacity building.

When systems prioritise scale without context, they weaken community agency. The result is a paradox where dominant health systems expand in reach while holistic well-being deteriorates.

The Need for Renewed Imagination

Confronting complex health challenges requires more than programmatic improvements; it demands renewed imagination. Co-design offers a pathway forward by enabling:

- Plurality rather than uniformity
- Dialogue rather than prescription
- Shared responsibility rather than dependency
- Evolution rather than replacement

This shift moves us from a model of delivery to one of partnership.

Understanding the Persistence of Health Challenges

Despite the rich cultural health foundation, several forces disrupt the functioning and transmission of traditional knowledge and contribute to persistent health inequities. These include:

1. Fragmentation between traditional and modern health systems, leading to mistrust and limited cross-learning.
2. Erosion of intergenerational knowledge transfer, accelerated by urban migration and cultural shifts.
3. Commercialisation and standardisation pressures, which convert community practices into decontextualised products rather than living traditions.
4. Lack of collaborative research frameworks, which restrict the ability to study and validate community-derived insights.
5. Rigid policy environments and institutional hierarchies, which often undervalue experiential or vernacular knowledge.
6. Rising chronic diseases, requiring holistic, sustained engagement rather than episodic medical intervention.

Together, these challenges point to a profound need for rethinking how knowledge is created, shared, and applied to health systems transformation.

A Call for Interdisciplinary Collaboration

To build future-ready rural health ecosystems, we must foster dialogue and co-creation among:

- Experts in health co-design and participatory innovation
- Traditional medicine and yoga practitioners working at community level
- Scholars and practitioners in rural development and social innovation
- Public health professionals and clinical experts
- Civil society organisations and frontline health workers
- Community leaders, elders, and youth

Collaborative health action must move beyond consultation into shared visioning, shared implementation, and shared ownership of outcomes. Participatory approaches can not only generate more meaningful and culturally appropriate interventions but also build trust, responsibility, and long-term sustainability.

Co-Learning and Co-Design for Chronic Health Challenges

To deepen this discussion, it is imperative to ground the concepts in lived realities. Health co-design is not an abstract philosophy—it is a practice that unfolds in the everyday lives of individuals and communities. The following narrative examples illustrate the power of participatory, context-aware approaches to managing chronic and complex health conditions.

Case Narrative 1: A Personal Journey with Diabetes (Real-Person Narrative)

Ramesh (name changed), a 52-year-old farmer from a semi-rural community, had lived with diabetes for nearly a decade. His condition worsened over time as medication routines became difficult to sustain and food practices shifted due to market availability and irregular work cycles. Conventional diabetes management advice felt disconnected from his lived realities: diet charts based on unfamiliar foods, rigid exercise prescriptions, and medical visits that addressed symptoms rather than daily life.

Through a community-led co-design initiative facilitated by local health workers and traditional practitioners, Ramesh joined a learning circle where community members, a yoga therapist, an Ayurveda practitioner, and a public health researcher engaged in open dialogue about diabetes. Rather than being instructed, participants shared experiences about how seasonal foods affected energy levels, how stress during crop failures impacted sugar fluctuations, and how morning yoga improved sleep and insulin sensitivity.

Together, the group co-created a personalised health plan integrating traditional millet-based foods from local agriculture, a collectively designed low-cost kitchen garden for medicinal herbs, and a daily 20-minute yoga routine suited to the rhythms of farm work. Peer support and community accountability proved transformative. Within months, Ramesh reported increased vitality, reduced medication dependency under medical supervision, and greater emotional resilience, saying: "I no longer feel alone in this. Health is a shared journey."

This example demonstrates how co-design can transform health from an individual medical struggle into a shared process of community empowerment.

Case Narrative 2: Designing a Community-Centric Health Response (System-Level Example)

In a rural district facing rising cases of diabetes and hypertension, local health officials initially relied on conventional public health strategies—awareness campaigns, screening drives, and distribution of printed informational materials. Despite high attendance, measurable improvements were limited, and follow-up engagement remained low.

Recognising the limitations of top-down approaches, the district shifted toward a co-design methodology. A series of participatory workshops brought together villagers, panchayat members, school teachers, youth groups, ASHA workers, yoga practitioners, and representatives of traditional medicine. Rather than starting with predefined solutions, the process began by listening: What barriers prevented people from managing chronic diseases? What strengths already existed within the community?

Key insights that emerged included the following:

- People were overwhelmed by conflicting advice from multiple health sources.
- Daily routines made consistent treatment difficult.
- Traditional food knowledge was declining, replaced by processed market foods.
- Community members trusted informal advice networks more than formal systems.

In response, the community co-developed an integrated model that combined weekly health circles hosted in common cultural spaces, training ASHA workers in dietary counselling using local foods, mobile yoga sessions for women in self-help groups, and locally created media in vernacular language featuring stories of community champions.

Outcomes included increases in follow-up compliance, improved blood sugar awareness, reduction in social stigma around chronic diseases, and greater trust in the health system. The most meaningful change was the emergence of a shared sense of responsibility—health became something done together rather than delivered to the community from outside.

These case narratives reinforce the principle that co-design creates impact not by importing solutions but by strengthening collective intelligence, shared ownership, and cultural alignment. Conditions such as diabetes illustrate the urgent need for integrative, community-anchored health strategies. Diabetes is not merely a biomedical condition; it is social, emotional, behavioural, and environmental. Effective management requires personalised pathways, community support, food literacy, accessibility, and emotional resilience. Co-design enables communities to collectively develop strategies that combine biomedical understanding with local food traditions, seasonal rhythms, yoga-based practice, and peer support networks.

Such collaborative approaches shift us from treating diseases to cultivating wellness.

Toward Participatory Health Innovation Models

Innovative health interventions created through participatory design may include:

- Community-led learning and healing circles
- Food and lifestyle interventions rooted in local biodiversity
- Integrative models combining AYUSH, yoga, and modern care
- Peer-led and youth-led health innovation platforms
- Low-cost frugal innovations emerging from lived experience
- Living labs that allow real-world experimentation and feedback

These models reposition communities from consumers to co-creators of health futures.

Building Collaborative Futures

A future-oriented approach to rural health transformation must nurture ecosystems rather than isolated projects. Co-design requires enabling environments where communities and institutions collaborate continuously, learning from one another and adapting to evolving contexts. The following pathways outline possibilities for long-term collaborative action:

Pathway 1. Creating Community-Based Learning and Innovation Networks

Networks of villages, health practitioners, educational institutions, NGOs, and local government bodies can serve as platforms for shared experimentation. Such networks enable cross-learning across diverse geographies, support documentation of traditional knowledge, and facilitate collective problem-solving. These learning ecosystems can become catalysts for frugal innovation, social entrepreneurship, and local resource mobilisation.

Pathway 2. Establishing Living Laboratories for Rural Health and Well-Being

Living laboratories provide real-world environments where solutions are co-designed, tested, and iteratively improved. They enable alignment between traditional health wisdom, modern research, and community priorities. A living lab approach encourages evidence creation that is participatory, contextualised, and grounded in everyday life rather than controlled laboratory conditions.

Pathway 3. Integrating Vernacular Health Knowledge with Modern Healthcare Models

Rather than viewing AYUSH and biomedical care as competing paradigms, future systems can facilitate synergy, i.e., leveraging the strengths of both. Yoga can complement clinical care; dietary interventions rooted in biodiversity can support metabolic health; and community-based psychosocial practices can strengthen resilience. Collaborative protocols and co-research models can generate evidence that honours multiple ways of knowing.

Pathway 4. Capacity Building and Training for Co-Design

To expand co-design adoption, practitioners—including public health workers, doctors, traditional healers, researchers, and students—can be trained in participatory facilitation, empathy-based inquiry, and collaborative innovation. Capacity-building initiatives can cultivate humility, listening, and shared decision-making as core competencies.

Pathway 5. Leveraging Education and Research Institutions as Bridges

Universities and research institutes can become connectors between communities, policymakers, and health practitioners. By shifting from transactional outreach to long-term partnership models, academic institutions can help co-generate knowledge rather than extract it. Participatory research frameworks and transdisciplinary engagement can expand the legitimacy of vernacular knowledge.

Pathway 6. Reimagining Policy and Governance Frameworks

Policy structures that recognise community agency and support distributed leadership can accelerate change. Policies must enable flexible funding, community research participation, indigenous knowledge protection, and multi-stakeholder governance.

Towards a Shared Future

The vision offered is not a blueprint but an invitation. Rural health transformation will emerge from many pathways, many voices, and many forms of wisdom in dialogue. Co-design provides the enabling architecture to weave these threads into a tapestry of shared purpose and collective well-being.

As we look to the future, may we cultivate:

- Curiosity instead of certainty
- Courage instead of caution
- Community instead of separation

Health is not a destination—it is a living practice, renewed each day through relationships of care.

Closing Reflection

This opening chapter is a call to reimagine what is possible when we learn together, design together, and heal together. It affirms that rural communities hold within them profound knowledge for living well and that the path to resilient, equitable health systems lies in partnership, humility, and shared imagination.

Let this monograph become a space of discovery, inspiration, and collective responsibility—a movement toward futures where well-being is co-created and belongs to all. The path ahead requires establishing networks and alliances that allow diverse stakeholders to continue learning and collaborating. Such networks can serve as platforms for:

- Sharing and synthesising knowledge across traditions
- Generating evidence collaboratively
- Supporting capacity building and training
- Creating policy frameworks that honour plurality
- Enabling scale without eroding cultural integrity

Conclusions

Health co-design invites us to reimagine the meaning of well-being and our collective responsibility in shaping futures of health. It calls upon us to move beyond the boundaries of our disciplines, professions, and inherited assumptions toward a more expansive and compassionate understanding of what it means to care. In doing so, it challenges us to listen, not only to data, institutions, or expert discourse but also to the wisdom embedded in everyday life, the voices of those who live closest to the challenges we seek to address, and the knowledge traditions that have nurtured communities for centuries.

If we believe that every community holds within it the intelligence required to flourish, then the task before us is not to deliver solutions but to create conditions where solutions can emerge. Co-design is an act of trust: trust that people know their lives better than anyone else; trust that meaningful change arises when power is shared; trust that learning together is more transformative than prescribing answers; trust that healing is not merely biological but relational, cultural, ecological, and spiritual.

In present times, when the world faces unprecedented health complexities—from chronic disease to mental distress, from environmental degradation to fragmented social systems—we must recognise that no single worldview, methodology, or institution possesses all the answers. The future of health lies in the ability to weave knowledge across traditions, disciplines, and generations. It lies in revitalising community agency and honouring the plurality of ways of knowing.

Imagine a future where health interventions are not imposed but co-created; where traditional healers and biomedical practitioners work side by side with mutual respect; where youth and elders collaborate in redefining what well-being means for their community; where the rhythms of the body, land, and society are once again aligned. Imagine a network of communities learning from one another, carrying forward stories of resilience, innovation, and shared transformation.

This monograph is offered in that spirit—an invitation to dream together, to design together, and to care together. May it serve as a seed for deeper collaboration and a reminder that collective imagination is one of our most powerful medicines.

The journey toward healthier communities begins with a simple, courageous act: to listen deeply, act together, and trust in the wisdom we already hold. The future of health is not something we wait for; it is something we co-create. Let us move forward with humility, hope, and the courage to imagine a world where well-being belongs to everyone.

Perspective 2

Community-Centred Ayurvedic Practices for Holistic Well-Being

Dr Chandrakant Desai
Traditional Vaidya, Yadgud

Background

Ayurveda has deep roots in community health as well as individual care. Its founding myth tells of sages praying for a universal healing system during a time of mass suffering. The classical aim of Ayurveda, as stated in the *Caraka Samhita,* is to "protect the health of the healthy and to cure diseases of the patient." In this framework, wellness means far more than the absence of illness; it includes mental balance, cultural traditions, and harmony with seasonal cycles. Modern observers note that many potent Ayurvedic practices continue in rural communities, even if mainstream science has not fully examined them. These community-based traditions, from healing rituals with natural elements to seasonal diets and life-cycle ceremonies, provide holistic, low-cost preventive care and can complement contemporary medicine.

Celestial Water Rituals

One notable practice is the collection and use of special waters believed to have healing qualities. For example, water gathered after the rising of the star Agastya (Canopus), called *Hamsodaka* or *Swatijala,* is traditionally considered exceptionally pure and rejuvenating. Families in parts of southern India preserve this water, drinking and using it for cooking and bathing throughout the year. Temples also collect it as a sacred *tirtha* offered to newborns and mothers. Some experts have suggested studying such water under different conditions (for example, comparing regions where Agastya is visible year-round to regions where it rises seasonally) to test these claims. In any case, these simple communal water rituals emphasise that health can be nurtured through everyday acts and reinforce the importance of public health.

Seasonal Dietary Regimens

Ayurveda emphasises aligning the diet with natural cycles. In spring (*Chaitra* season), people traditionally consume neem leaves and flowers for their purifying and cooling effect. Rather than a single-day remedy, this is a full-season regimen. One related practice is the consumption of *Chaitra Churna,* a powdered blend of seasonal herbs, daily throughout spring. Practitioners report noticeable benefits at very low cost: reduced body heat, clearer skin, and improved digestion.

Similarly, at the onset of the monsoon (during *Mriga Nakshatra,* roughly June 6–15 each year), communities once ate drumstick tree (Moringa) leaf dishes frequently. Moringa leaves are mildly alkaline and nutrient-rich, helping to balance the acidity of the rainy season. Today, this practice has largely faded to a single-day observance, but it reflects a deep understanding of preventive nutrition through local foods.

Beyond specific herbs, traditional dietary wisdom prescribes the use of all six tastes (*shadrasa*) in every meal. A balanced plate would include: sweet foods (e.g., rice) to support stability (*Kapha*), followed by sour and salty items for balance (supporting Kapha and *Pitta*), and pungent, bitter, and astringent foods at the end (to balance Pitta and *Vata*).

This sequence corresponds to traditional concepts of the body's elements (*doshas*). For example, starting a meal with something sweet may help build vitality (Kapha), while ending with bitter or astringent spices supports digestive balance. In short, including all six tastes in each meal is believed to maintain harmony among the body's elements.

Early-Life Rituals and Infant Nutrition

Early-life rituals (*samskaras*) are considered essential

for lifelong health. Within moments of birth, simple ceremonies prepare an infant's senses. For instance, a pair of small pebbles is gently tapped near the baby's ear (right ear for boys, left for girls). This soft, natural sound is said to connect the newborn to the pure element of space (*akasa*) and initiate hearing in a calm way. Naming ceremonies (*Namakarana*) follow astrological guidelines (birth star and gender). Each child receives both an everyday name and a sacred name drawn from revered figures. These names carry blessings and symbolic protection.

Key infant rites include *Karnavedana* (ear piercing) and *Nasavedana* (nose piercing). These rituals are viewed not merely as ornamental but as methods to bolster immunity, vitality, and future reproductive health. (They are performed at a young age, somewhat like early vaccination, to confer long-term protection.) In traditional communities, breastfeeding is viewed as a sacred duty. A mother's milk (*stanya*) is revered as "living medicine". It serves not only as the infant's first food but also as a remedy for childhood coughs, asthma, digestive issues, and eye conditions. If a mother cannot nurse, Ayurveda advises selecting a *dhātrī* (wet nurse) whose health and constitution closely match the baby's, ensuring the substitute milk is as nourishing as possible. This practice reflects an early form of personalised nutrition.

Small amounts of gentle herbal mixtures are given as supplements to newborn infants. One example is

Balaguti—selected herbs rubbed with water or honey, offered to infants between about 10 days and two years of age.

These home-prepared tonics have been used for generations, acting as mild health-promoting remedies without harsh side effects.

These practices illustrate how Ayurveda weaves nutrition and care into a child's earliest days, emphasising gentle support over chemical intervention.

Everyday Preventive Practices

Daily life in Ayurvedic communities also includes simple health practices using readily available materials. One well-known example is *kajal* (kohl). Carefully prepared at home from soot and herbs, kajal is not merely a cosmetic; it is believed to cleanse, strengthen, and soothe the eyes. For centuries, mothers and sisters have applied a thin line of kajal on young children's eyelids to ward off irritation or infection. Even today, some elders still prepare kajal by hand and use it as an eye remedy.

Other commonplace items serve a preventive role.

Protective jewellery: The tiny metal *kudakū* stud worn in the ear by some tribal women has been associated (anecdotally) with lower rates of breast and uterine cancer. This might be due to contact with an acupuncture-like point in the ear or a trace-metal effect, but in any case, it highlights a practical approach to protection.

Amulets and bracelets: Families often give infants

simple charms or woollen bands. For example, a fine woollen bracelet tied around a baby's wrist or ankle acts as a dust trap. In dusty environments, the fibres capture particulate matter before it reaches the child's lungs. Parents report fewer coughs in children who wear such woollen traps. Similarly, charms made of animal parts (tiger teeth, deer skin, etc.) or special beads are kept for traditional protective value.

These everyday talismans and remedies embody a folk logic of health: using what is at hand to protect the body. Together with household medicine (like herbal teas), they reinforce the principle that health can largely be maintained at home.

Ghee as Medicine and Food

No account of traditional Ayurvedic practice is complete without *ghee* (*ghrta*). Ghee is clarified butter, but in Ayurveda, it is treated as both food and medicine. Classical texts list 16 special qualities of ghee and note that it embodies all six tastes, making it *tridoṣhic* (balancing to all constitutions). Fresh homemade ghee is valued for daily cooking and digestion, while aged ghee (*purana* ghrta) is considered especially potent.

Ageing ghee can increase its medicinal properties. Some families keep jars of ghee for decades. One well-known example is a jar of 75-year-old ghee that is applied to chronic wounds or even ingested for slow-healing fractures. In many such cases, patients who had not responded well to modern treatments have improved with careful ghee therapy. Pilgrimage traditions also reflect these beliefs: at Srisailam, devotees pour fresh ghee into rocky potholes along the temple path. Over time, the ghee darkens and is believed to absorb minerals. Pilgrims collect this rock-aged ghee on their return journey, confident that it can heal minor ailments.

Ghee is also used in special preparations. A tiny amount of water that naturally collects in *desi* ghee (*ghrtamanda*) is taken for relief from migraine. *Ksirasarpi,* ghee made directly from milk rather than from fermented butter, is traditionally used for gynecological health complaints.

In general, ghee is prescribed to soothe inflammation, lubricate joints, and rejuvenate tissues. The Ayurvedic emphasis on ageing ghee (for example, *kumbhaghrta* is 100-year-old ghee, *mahaghrta* is over 100 years old) underscores the belief that time enhances its potency. With good reason, ghee is often cited as an ideal example of a substance that fully nourishes the body with virtually no adverse effects.

Conclusions

The examples above illustrate the rich practical wisdom of Ayurvedic tradition as it is lived in communities. They highlight that health in these societies is understood as seasonal, cultural, and woven into daily life. Many of the remedies and rituals described have never been disproven by science; instead, they await systematic investigation. Dismissing them out of hand ignores generations of observation. Instead, there is a strong case for integration—investigating these practices with modern tools while respecting indigenous knowledge.

Reviving such traditions need not mean rejecting contemporary medicine. Rather, it offers complementary, low-cost paths that are culturally familiar and aligned with natural rhythms. The ultimate goal, as Ayurveda teaches, is *swasthya*—complete well-being for individuals, families, and the entire community. By remembering and honouring traditional wisdom in everyday actions, through the water used, the foods eaten, the rites performed, and even the ghee in the kitchen, health, in the broadest sense, is nurtured. Community well-being depends as much on these time-tested home remedies and rituals as on modern clinics and hospitals.

References

Arora, V. (2025). "Hansodhak: An Ayurvedic perspective of water purification in Sharad Ritu with modern correlation". *AYUSHDHARA*, 12(4), 303–310.

Bhavamishra. (2015). "*Bhavaprakasha Nighantu* (Ghrita Varga)". In K. C. Chunekar (Ed.) & G. S. Pandey (Trans.), *Bhavaprakasha Nighantu: Indian materia medica.* Chaukhamba Bharati Academy.

Pandey, D. et al. (2022). "Formulation and evaluation of medicated herbal kajal". *International Journal of Scientific Research in Science and Technology*, 9(3), 603–609.

Pandey, R. B. (1969). *Hindu Saṃskāras: Socio-religious study of the Hindu sacraments* (2nd rev. ed.). Motilal Banarsidass Publishers.

Patwardhan, B., Warude, D., Pushpangadan, P., & Bhatt, N. (2005). "Ayurveda and traditional Chinese medicine: A comparative overview". *Evidence-Based Complementary and Alternative Medicine,* 2(4), 465–473.

Sharma, P. V. (Trans.). (2014). *Charaka Samhita: Text with English translation.* Chaukhambha Orientalia.

World Health Organization. (2013). *WHO traditional medicine strategy: 2014–2023.*

Perspective 3

Does Ayurveda have Solutions for Extreme Events such as the Pandemic? Experiences from COVID-19

Dr P. L. T. Girija

Sanjeevani Ayurveda and Yoga Centre

Adyar, Chennai

Introduction

The COVID-19 pandemic posed an unprecedented challenge to global health systems. Faced with a novel pathogen and limited therapeutic clarity, public health infrastructures across the world were forced into reactive modes of care. In India, the dominant response framework was shaped by modern biomedicine, with central institutions such as the Indian Council of Medical Research, All India Institute of Medical Sciences, and

Postgraduate Institute of Medical Education and Research, guiding protocols and policy.

Within this landscape, a critical question emerged: Could Ayurveda, India's classical medical system, offer a viable response to a pandemic of this magnitude? The practitioner perspective presented here argues in the affirmative. It documents clinical experiences of standalone Ayurvedic management of COVID-19 across mild, moderate, severe, and high-risk categories, including patients with multiple co-morbidities. Beyond clinical outcomes, it reflects on the future health preparedness of Ayurveda and the need for a change in public health policy.

Epidemics in Ayurvedic Thought: *Janapadodhwamsa*

Ayurveda is not unfamiliar with the concept of epidemic diseases. The classical text *Charaka Samhita* describes *janapadodhwamsa*—the large-scale affliction or destruction of communities due to disturbances in air, water, land, and seasonal rhythms. This framework, articulated in foundational treatises, recognises that when ecological and environmental balance is disturbed, it gives rise to epidemic disease. During epidemics, even otherwise healthy individuals are susceptible.

The Ayurvedic texts provide extensive elaboration on *jwara* (fever), which occupies a central position in Ayurvedic nosology. Fever is analysed not as a monolithic condition but as a spectrum of pathologies arising from various combinations of vata, pitta, and kapha (doshas), involving different tissues (*dhatus*), organ systems, and psychological states. Acute, chronic, intermittent, traumatic, emotional, and systemic fevers are described in detail, along with their etiologies, symptomatology, dietetic guidance, regimens, and therapeutic approaches.

Ayurvedic practitioners, who are experienced in managing viral fevers such as dengue, chikungunya, and influenza-like illnesses, approached COVID-19 as a novel manifestation within an established diagnostic grammar rather than as an incomprehensible anomaly. From the early cases of COVID-19, clinical presentations were diagnosed as vata-kapha jwara, enabling therapeutic direction grounded in textual precedent.

Clinical Practice under Constraint

Despite Ayurveda's theoretical preparedness, institutional acceptance was limited. In several regions, official sanction for independent Ayurvedic management of COVID-19 was either absent or actively discouraged. In Tamil Nadu, attempts were made to collaborate formally with biomedical authorities; however, proposed clinical trials required Ayurveda to function adjunctively, restricting prescriptions to single drugs alongside allopathic medicines and treatments. This placed severe restrictions on ayurvedic treatment protocols for COVID-19.

In the absence of any official mandate, treatment was undertaken on an outpatient basis under home quarantine. A standardised case record format later issued by the Ministry of AYUSH facilitated systematic documentation, including demographic data, co-morbidities, symptom progression, consent, and daily monitoring parameters.

Inclusion criteria were straightforward: patients opting exclusively for Ayurvedic treatment. Those seeking simultaneous allopathic and ayurvedic interventions were excluded as it was a standalone ayurvedic treatment. As no institutional admission privileges were granted for Ayurvedic hospitals for COVID-positive patients, even a functioning 40-bed hospital could not be utilised, and all care occurred remotely through carefully monitored home-based protocols.

Daily teleconsultations formed the backbone of management. Patients were guided to self-monitor fever, appetite, bowel movements, respiratory effort, cough severity, fatigue, and general orientation. Although oxygen saturation (SpO_2) was not traditionally central to Ayurvedic assessment, it became part of practical monitoring due to public familiarity with pulse oximeter during the pandemic. Clinical decisions, however, were guided by symptom clusters and progression patterns consistent with Ayurvedic diagnostics.

Treatment Protocol and Therapeutic Rationale

A compact therapeutic kit was developed, typically comprising selected *kashayams* (decoctions), *churnas* (powders), and tablets. These were adapted case-by-case. More than 90 per cent of cases were managed using a core set of formulations, with additional medicines introduced when needed.

In instances of persistent cough and breathlessness (*shwasa-kasa*), the principle of *muhur muhur*—frequent, repeated administration of medicines in small doses—was employed, and patients were instructed to consume measured quantities at hourly or bi-hourly intervals during waking hours. *Rasayana* (rejuvenative) formulations were prescribed during recovery to restore vitality and systemic resilience.

Metal- and mineral-based formulations were used sparingly and judiciously, and contrary to common perceptions, no adverse hepatic or renal outcomes were observed in documented cases. The pharmacological rationale followed classical guidelines concerning dosage, *anupana* (vehicle), and constitution of patients.

Clinical Data and Outcomes

Across three waves of the pandemic, 781 documented cases were treated. An additional number, estimated to exceed 1,000, were managed informally during the earliest months before systematic documentation was established.

Of the documented cohort, 419 were female and 362 were male. One hundred and eighty-four patients were above 60 years of age; 124 had diabetes; 113 had hypertension; 46 had asthma; 11 had cancer; 15 had chronic kidney disease; and 8 had chronic obstructive pulmonary disease. Out of 540 patients with co-morbidities, 81 had multiple co-morbidities. Thirty-four were asymptomatic; the majority presented with respiratory symptoms, often accompanied by fatigue, fever, sore throat, diarrhoea, and myalgia.

Recovery time averaged approximately six days (± 2 days), with younger patients typically recovering more rapidly. Even severe cases presenting with hypoxemia—oxygen saturation in the 70s—were managed under home quarantine using intensive monitoring and muhur muhur dosing. Deterioration during Ayurvedic management was not observed within this documented cohort.

Three fatalities occurred. The first was a 78-year-old outstation patient who received the medication late in the disease course and passed away shortly thereafter. The second was an 88-year-old male who was bedridden with severe dementia and multiple co-morbidities and could not communicate with treating doctors. The third fatality was a double-vaccinated 85-year-old male. He was a heart patient with COPD and reduced kidney function. He was being treated for COVID-19 with steroids and paracetamol. The inclusion of these patients reflected compassionate grounds rather than ideal eligibility criteria. These cases were transparently recorded.

The overall treatment cost for the entire duration—from first consultation to resolution—was approximately Rs. 3,000 per patient, including medicines and follow-up.

Illustrative High-Risk Cases

Several high-risk cases highlight the scope of intervention. A 57-year-old woman with longstanding diabetes, hypertension, coronary artery disease, chronic kidney disease requiring thrice-weekly dialysis, chronic obstructive pulmonary disease, and a breast lesion recovered from COVID-19 under Ayurvedic management. Despite missing three dialysis sessions during active infection, her biochemical parameters remained stable; chest imaging showed no pulmonary deterioration. She later tested negative for COVID-19 by RT-PCR.

Other cases included cancer patients undergoing chemotherapy or radiation, elderly individuals with prior coronary artery bypass grafting, and patients with significant hypoxemia. In one instance, a patient in an intensive care setting of an allopathic hospital received Ayurvedic medication (details of administration logistics remain unclear) and reported rapid recovery.

Retrospective Reflections

From a retrospective perspective, several features stand out. First, there was no single universal Ayurvedic drug for COVID-19. Different practitioners employed varied formulations consistent with shared diagnostic principles. This pluralism reflects the strength of Ayurveda's case-based, constitution-sensitive methodology rather than a one-size-fits-all pharmaceutical model. More importantly, Ayurveda is able to treat a new disease with ease at a miniscule cost compared to modern Western medical care.

Second, symptom resolution was typically rapid, and disease progression was arrested early. Third, treatment proved economically accessible. Finally, mortality within the documented cohort was low relative to the severity and co-morbidity burden of patients treated.

The experience invites a broader policy question. India has more than 400,000 registered Ayurvedic practitioners. Had this human resource been systematically mobilised within public health planning, could community-level disease management have been more effective, decentralised, and decongested? The experience of traditional Chinese medicine's formal inclusion during the early COVID-19 response in China suggests that integrative approaches are institutionally feasible.

Ayurveda and Future Public Health Preparedness

Ayurveda conceptualises new diseases through the lens of recurring dosha dynamics rather than unique pathogens alone. When aggravated, one dosha can cause many different diseases. The treating physician is expected to comprehend the nature of the disease (dosha), the site of manifestation, and etiological factors and accordingly initiate treatment for any new disease.

Whether or not Ayurveda is adopted as the primary system of medical care, its conceptual resources for epidemic management and cost-effective care merit serious scholarly and policy engagement.

Conclusions

The COVID-19 pandemic revealed vulnerabilities in global health systems, but it also opened space for re-evaluating indigenous medical traditions. This practitioner account suggests that Ayurveda possesses conceptual frameworks, cost-effective therapeutic strategies, and community-level scalability, relevant to extreme public health events.

The central question is no longer whether Ayurveda can respond to pandemics in principle but whether future public health planning will meaningfully engage with its human and intellectual capital.

Perspective 4

Homeopathy for Health: A Collaborative Path to Personalised Wellness

Hardik Khamar
Homeopathy Care Clinics, Ahmedabad

Personalisation and the Search for Whole-Person Care

Recent developments in global healthcare discourse have renewed attention to personalised medicine and wellness. While technological advances in genomics, diagnostics, and data-driven medicine have shaped this conversation, the underlying concern—how to treat individuals rather than diseases—has a much longer intellectual history. Philosophical traditions from classical antiquity onwards have emphasised that health cannot be understood through isolated organs or symptoms alone but must be approached as an integrated state of physical, mental, and social balance.

Homoeopathy is situated within this lineage of whole-person care. Its foundational premise holds that health is not merely the absence of disease but a dynamic equilibrium within the individual. From this perspective, treatment aims not only at symptom relief but also at restoring balance across bodily, emotional, and adaptive dimensions of health. This paper explores how such an approach resonates with contemporary calls for collaborative and personalised healthcare.

Homoeopathy and the Idea of Personalised Medicine

The concept of personalised medicine has gained prominence in recent years, particularly within biomedical research institutions and policy forums. Typically associated with precision diagnostics and targeted therapies, personalisation is often framed in technological terms. However, traditional medical systems—including homoeopathy, Ayurveda, and other knowledge traditions—have long operationalised personalisation through detailed patient narratives, contextual histories, and individualised therapeutic responses.

Homoeopathy is explicitly founded on the principle that no two individuals experience illness in identical ways. Therapeutic decisions are, therefore, based on the totality of symptoms, encompassing physical complaints, emotional states, behavioural patterns, and life circumstances. This approach resists standardised, one-size-fits-all protocols and instead adopts what may be described as a "cafeteria" model of care, in which interventions are selected and sequenced according to individual need.

Such an orientation positions homoeopathy as a potential collaborator within integrative healthcare models, particularly in contexts where chronic illness, lifestyle disorders, and post-infectious conditions demand long-term, adaptive care rather than acute intervention alone.

Post-Pandemic Context and the Need for Integrative Health Systems

The COVID-19 pandemic has been described as a period of sustained global disruption, marked by prolonged uncertainty, systemic stress, and widespread health consequences extending beyond acute infection. The emergence of long COVID and associated psychosocial impacts has further challenged conventional healthcare delivery models.

In this context, integrative healthcare has gained renewed relevance. Collaboration between biomedical and traditional systems offers opportunities to address not only physiological recovery but also emotional resilience, social reintegration, and adaptive coping. Homoeopathy's emphasis on individual narratives and long-term follow-up aligns with these needs, particularly in managing post-pandemic fatigue, metabolic imbalance, and stress-related conditions.

Case Illustrations from Clinical Practice

Clinical practice across diverse settings demonstrates how homoeopathy can be part of a collaborative, personalised care framework.

In one instance, an adult patient developed hypertension and metabolic imbalance following COVID-19 infection, accompanied by obesity, fatigue, emotional isolation, and psychosocial stress. Homoeopathic intervention focused on the individual's overall physical and emotional profile rather than blood pressure values alone. Over time, blood pressure stabilised within normal limits, alongside improvements in weight regulation, emotional well-being, and self-esteem. This case highlights the importance of addressing post-infectious illness holistically.

Another illustration involved a child experiencing *alopecia universalis* following severe emotional trauma. Treatment was guided by the child's psychological state, behavioural changes, and life context. Over a sustained follow-up period, hair regrowth was accompanied by social reintegration, return to schooling, and emotional recovery. The outcome underscored the importance of addressing grief and trauma as integral components of physical illness.

Further cases from urban practice demonstrated the supportive role of homoeopathy in complex conditions such as cancer survivorship and neurological disorders. In patients undergoing conventional treatment for serious illness, homoeopathy served as an adjunct to mitigate treatment-related side effects, enhance emotional resilience, and improve quality of life. In paediatric neurodevelopmental conditions, collaborative engagement with occupational therapy, behavioural interventions, and educational support proved essential, reinforcing the value of multidisciplinary care.

Across these cases, the central feature was not disease-specific cure but restoration of functional capacity, emotional stability, and adaptive balance over time.

Collaboration, Empathy, and the Role of the Patient

A defining characteristic of homoeopathic practice is the depth of patient engagement. Detailed case-taking emphasises empathy, attentive listening, and systematic documentation of lived experience. This process positions the patient as an active collaborator in care rather than a passive recipient of treatment.

Empathy, in this context, is understood not as emotional over-identification but as structured attentiveness that informs clinical decision-making while maintaining professional boundaries. Such an approach enables practitioners to integrate subjective narratives with objective observation, supporting personalised prescription and long-term monitoring.

Community engagement further extends this collaborative model. In both rural and urban contexts, trust-building, continuity of care, and patient education play critical roles in sustaining therapeutic relationships and facilitating health literacy.

Challenges of Standardisation and Evidence

Despite its potential contributions, homoeopathy faces significant challenges within contemporary healthcare systems. The individualised nature of treatment complicates conventional models of standardisation, measurement, and randomised controlled trials. While outcome documentation and long-term follow-up can provide valuable practice-based evidence, methodological frameworks capable of capturing individualised interventions remain underdeveloped.

These challenges underscore the need for innovative evaluation strategies that respect the epistemological foundations of personalised care while meeting ethical and scientific standards. Integrative health systems must, therefore, balance flexibility with accountability, and innovation with patient safety.

Practice Implications for Health Co-Design

The experiences outlined in this paper suggest several implications for health co-design. Homoeopathy is particularly well-suited to primary healthcare contexts, chronic disease management, and conditions requiring sustained psychosocial engagement. Its integration within broader health systems is most effective when framed as complementarity rather than substitution.

Health co-design benefits from recognising multiple therapeutic logics and enabling collaborative referral pathways. Technology, including digital record-keeping and outcome tracking, can support this process without undermining individualised care. Ultimately, co-designed health systems must prioritise wellness creation over disease management alone.

Lessons for Integrating Homoeopathy in Personalised Healthcare:

- Individualised treatment is central to effective personalised care.
- Empathy and structured case-taking enhance clinical insight and patient trust.
- Homeopathy functions most effectively as a complementary modality within integrative systems.
- Long-term follow-up and documentation are essential for ethical practice.
- Collaborative engagement with other health disciplines strengthens outcomes.

Positioning Within the Health Co-Design Discourse

This chapter contributes a practice-led perspective to the health co-design discourse by illustrating how personalised, empathetic, and integrative care unfolds in real-world clinical settings. It complements conceptual and policy-oriented discussions within this volume by demonstrating how homoeopathy can participate responsibly in collaborative health systems.

By foregrounding lived experience, patient partnership, and ethical reflexivity, the chapter underscores the relevance of traditional systems of medicine in addressing contemporary health challenges, particularly in contexts demanding long-term, person-centred care.

References

Goodman, M. L., Molldrem, S., Elliott, A., Robertson, D., & Keiser, P. (2023). "Long COVID and mental health correlates: A new chronic condition fits existing patterns". *Health Psychology and Behavioral Medicine,* 11(1), 2164498.

Hahnemann, S. (1842/1921). *Organon of Medicine* (6th ed.). (J. Künzli, A. Naudé, & P. Pendleton, Trans.). Victor Gollancz.

Halpern, J. (2003). "What is clinical empathy?" *Journal of General Internal Medicine,* 18(8), 670–674.

Hamburg, M. A. & Collins, F. S. (2010). "The path to personalized medicine". *New England Journal of Medicine,* 363(4), 301–304.

Institute for Healthcare Improvement. (2023). *The evolution of patient-centered care and the meaning of co-design.*

World Health Organization. (2025). *WHO global traditional medicine strategy 2025–2034.*

Perspective 5

How Self-Care Practices Can Improve Overall Individual Well-Being

Purnima Arun
Sehat Aur Swad
Ghaziabad

Background

Contemporary health systems face increasing strain due to rising chronic disease burdens, unequal access to care, and growing dependence on institutional medical services for conditions that are often preventable or manageable at the household and community level. This paper examines the role of self-care practices in enhancing overall individual well-being, drawing on experiential knowledge rooted in household traditions, community practices, and principles aligned with Ayurveda. Rather than positioning self-care as an alternative to modern medicine, the paper frames it as a complementary foundation for everyday health maintenance, prevention, and resilience. Through reflective illustrations from community-based practice, the paper argues that reviving context-specific, seasonal, and constitution-sensitive self-care practices can strengthen individual agency, reduce medical dependence, and contribute meaningfully to health co-design.

Reclaiming Self-Care in Contemporary Health Systems

Health discourse in recent decades has increasingly focused on institutional care, specialised treatment, and technological intervention. While these advances are essential for acute and critical conditions, they have also contributed to a gradual erosion of everyday health practices traditionally sustained within households and communities. In many societies, particularly in India, everyday self-care once formed the first line of health maintenance, with families relying on food practices, behavioural discipline, and seasonal routines to sustain well-being.

This paper explores how such self-care practices—often transmitted informally across generations—can be re-articulated within contemporary health co-design frameworks. It argues that self-care is not a regression to the past but a necessary response to the limitations of health systems that cannot feasibly reach every individual for every minor ailment.

Household Knowledge and the Foundations of Health

Historically, household practices related to cooking, feeding, and daily routines functioned as embedded health systems. Knowledge regarding what to eat, when to eat, how much to eat, and what to avoid was shaped by close observation of seasons, local biodiversity, and individual constitution. Such knowledge was rarely codified in formal texts, yet it was systematically transmitted through practice, observation, and social learning.

These practices emphasised the freshness of food, its digestibility and alignment with climate and bodily needs, as well as moderation. Minor ailments such as colds, digestive disturbances, or skin conditions were commonly managed at home, while external medical intervention was sought primarily for severe or acute conditions. This layered approach to care reduced unnecessary medical dependence and cultivated confidence in self-regulation of health.

Modernisation, Medicalisation, and the Loss of Self-Reliance

The processes of modernisation and urbanisation, as well as changing family structures have significantly disrupted traditional self-care systems. Nuclear households, reduced intergenerational contact, and time-scarce lifestyles have weakened everyday transmission of health knowledge. Simultaneously, expanding medical infrastructure and increased availability of pharmaceuticals have normalised seeking professional intervention for even minor discomforts.

This shift has contributed to a culture of over-medicalisation, where individuals often perceive health as something managed externally by doctors, hospitals, and diagnostic tests. In such a framework, subjective well-being, emotional balance, and functional vitality receive less attention than numerical indicators and laboratory values. The erosion of self-care thus represents not only a loss of practical knowledge but also a narrowing of how health itself is understood.

Principles of Self-Care: Diet, Behaviour, and Mental Balance

Self-care practices articulated through household wisdom and Ayurvedic principles emphasise the interdependence of diet, behaviour, and mental state. Health is understood as a dynamic balance rather than a static condition. Dietary practices focus on seasonal appropriateness, simplicity, moderation, and digestibility. Behavioural discipline, including regular routines, adequate rest, and mindful engagement with work, supports physiological balance.

Equally central is mental and emotional regulation. Excessive anger, stress, and irritation are recognised as contributors to bodily imbalance, particularly affecting digestion and metabolic processes. Cultivating patience, calmness, and emotional restraint is, therefore, considered integral to health maintenance. In this view, self-care extends beyond physical practices to include ethical and emotional self-regulation.

Fasting or dietary restraint, when applied judiciously, is also regarded as a powerful restorative practice. A temporary reduction in intake allows physiological systems to recalibrate and recover, reinforcing the principle that less intervention can sometimes produce greater balance.

Illustrations from Community-Based Practice

Community-based experiences provide insight into the potential impact of self-care practices. Simple, locally known dietary preparations have been observed to improve nutritional status among children within short periods, reflected in visible markers such as energy levels and physical appearance. In other instances, individuals managing lifestyle-related conditions reported reduced dependence on long-term medication following sustained changes in diet and daily routines.

Women experiencing reproductive health challenges have similarly benefitted from constitution-sensitive dietary and behavioural adjustments, sometimes after prolonged engagement with high-intensity biomedical interventions. In such cases, self-care did not replace medical oversight but complemented it by addressing underlying metabolic and emotional imbalances.

These illustrations do not suggest universal outcomes or guaranteed cures. Instead, they demonstrate how self-care can function as a supportive and preventive framework that enhances resilience, recovery, and quality of life when practised consistently and contextually.

Self-Care, Faith, and Personal Agency

An often-overlooked dimension of self-care is the role of belief, confidence, and personal agency. Trust in one's capacity to actively participate in health maintenance can, in turn, influence outcomes by reinforcing adherence, patience, and long-term commitment. Faith, in this context, is not understood as blind belief but as experiential confidence developed through observation and practice.

Self-care practices foster a sense of empowerment, reducing fear and helplessness associated with illness. Individuals who understand the basic principles of diet, routine, and mental balance are better equipped to respond calmly to everyday health fluctuations, reserving institutional care for situations that genuinely require it.

Implications for Health Co-Design

From a health co-design perspective, self-care represents a foundational layer of the health ecosystem. Designing effective health systems requires recognising households and communities as active sites of care rather than passive recipients of services. Training community-based health facilitators or coaches can help translate traditional self-care knowledge into contemporary contexts while remaining sensitive to regional diversity.

Importantly, self-care should not be framed in opposition to modern medicine. Emergencies, critical illnesses, and complex conditions clearly require specialised medical intervention. However, strengthening self-care practices can reduce unnecessary burden on health systems, lower medical costs, and improve overall well-being.

Core Principles of Self-Care for Individual Well-Being:

- Alignment of diet with season, constitution, and climate
- Preference for freshly prepared, simple, and digestible foods
- Practice of moderation in intake and routine
- Attention to emotional balance and cultivation of patience
- Judicious use of fasting or dietary restraint when appropriate

Positioning Within the Health Co-Design Discourse

This chapter contributes a community- and household-centred perspective to the health co-design discourse. It complements clinical, institutional, and policy-oriented chapters in this volume by highlighting the often-overlooked role of everyday practices in sustaining health.

By foregrounding self-care as a shared responsibility between individuals, families, and health systems, the paper underscores the importance of restoring balance between institutional care and personal agency. In plural and resource-constrained contexts, such an approach is essential for building resilient, inclusive, and sustainable health systems.

References

Bandura, A. (1997). *Self-efficacy: The exercise of control.* W. H. Freeman and Company.

Bhatt, Y. & Kulshrestha, K. (2020). "What's in the kitchen: Conventional household practices during minor health problems". *European Journal of Nutrition & Food Safety*, 12(12), 104–111.

Charaka Samhita, "Sutrasthana", Chapter 6 (Tasyashiteeya Adhyaya – Seasonal Regimen). In: Sharma, P. V. (Trans.). (2014). *Charaka Samhita: Text with English translation.* Chaukhambha Orientalia.

Gu, L., Fu, R., Hong, J., Ni, H., Yu, K., & Lou, H. (2024). "Intermittent fasting and health outcomes: An umbrella review of systematic reviews and meta-analyses of randomised controlled trials". *eClinicalMedicine*, 70, 102519.

Illich, I. (1976). *Limits to medicine – Medical nemesis: The expropriation of health.* Marion Boyars Publishers.

Joshi, S., Bisht, A., Juyal, R., Sharma, R., & Gupta, A. (2021). "'Old is gold': How traditional Indian dietary practices can support healthy eating". *Nutrients,* 13(12), 4521.

Lad, V. (2002). *Textbook of Ayurveda: Fundamental principles.* The Ayurvedic Press.

Mathpati, M. M., Albert, S., & Porter, J. D. H. (2020). "Ayurveda and medicalisation today: The loss of important knowledge and practice in health?" *Journal of Ayurveda and Integrative Medicine,* 11(1), 89–94.

Shivanand, B. S., Tushara, M., Unnikrishnan, P. M., & Krishnamurthy, J. (2022). "Do integrative approaches to health contribute to self-reliance in primary healthcare? Reflections from a community case study in Kerala, India". *Health Psychology and Behavioral Medicine,* 10(1), 1124–1135.

World Health Organization. (2024, April 25). *Self-care for health and well-being* [Fact sheet].

Perspective 6

Integrative Healthcare and Community Wellness: A Health Co-Design Framework for "Seeing with Both Eyes"

Rashmi Raut Gadgil
Anandi Chikitsalay
Ajra, Maharashtra

Introduction

Healthcare in rural regions cannot be treated simply as a scaled-down version of urban medicine. It is a distinct field demanding preventive outreach and continuous care within resource-constrained settings. A focus on episodic treatment or symptom control is typically insufficient for long-term community well-being. The rapid spread of modern lifestyles, characterised by fast food, fast-paced living, and the notion that "newest is best", has often come at the cost of synchronisation with natural rhythms. Many rural families have shifted away from locally grown, nutritious foods toward processed, market-based diets, losing traditional dietary and lifestyle practices (*Ahara-Vihara*). Additionally, younger people are migrating to cities, leaving elders in isolated households. In cases of minor ailments, these elders may be unable to rest and recover from daily labour, creating pressure for quick fixes. For example, it is common to see elderly patients treated repeatedly with steroid injections or analgesics for arthritis. These "magic pills" bring immediate relief, but over the years, they can cause osteoporosis, kidney damage, cardiovascular problems, and lifelong medication dependence. When such a patient later consults an integrative doctor, tapering the steroid triggers severe pain and resistance, illustrating that clinical care fails when it stops at prescriptions alone. In this context, modern medicine, a byproduct of modernity, remains essential for acute care and emergencies but often struggles with complex, lifestyle-driven chronic illnesses. No single system is perfect. The framework proposed here acknowledges the strengths of each medicine system and seeks to use them appropriately to improve patient outcomes.

Integrative Healthcare and Co-design Framework

The core principle of the proposed model is metaphorically described as "seeing with both eyes". This does not mean indiscriminately blending systems, since modern biomedicine and traditional medicine have different philosophies. Instead, the guiding idea is to use the best of each system where appropriate. Modern medical science, with its rigorous diagnostics and well-defined protocols, excels at managing acute crises and emergencies. Traditional systems, by contrast, emphasise prevention, lifestyle regulation, and harmony with nature. For instance, simple Ayurvedic remedies or recognition of local medicinal plants (such as using Vasaka for asthma) can empower patients to care for themselves with the resources at hand. Traditional diagnostic approaches (like *darshan chikitsa,* or assessment by observation) can sometimes identify health risks early without costly tests. By judiciously combining these methods, the integrative practitioner can often reduce unnecessary medications, lower the need for expensive investigations, and prevent future complications.

Family medicine provides the practical foundation for this integrative model. A family physician's broad training (across internal medicine, pediatrics, obstetrics, etc.) and continuous relationship with patients enables early risk identification, repeated counselling, and holistic care. In rural contexts where specialist referral may be difficult, this generalist approach is crucial. The model adds a second component, "health co-design", which holds that health originates largely in daily life and domestic environments rather than solely in clinics. Stable habits and local food systems form the primary preventive layer. In today's fast-paced world, convenient packaged and processed foods have become ubiquitous, but these often contain unhealthy trans fats and additives. In contrast, freshly prepared home-cooked meals using locally available ingredients (chosen with attention to each person's constitution, or prakriti) have significant positive effects on family wellness. By promoting traditional diets and cooking with care, communities build resilience to non-communicable diseases and reduce dependence on medical interventions.

Health co-design also means involving communities as active participants in their care. Rather than imposing solutions, practitioners collaborate with patients, families, local healers, and other stakeholders to identify needs and develop interventions. For example, an urban family migrated to a rural area, built a traditional clay home using cow-dung plaster, and planned their diet around seasonal, locally grown foods. This household became a venue for co-design: the kitchen, daily routines, and home remedies were organised to align with natural rhythms and agricultural cycles. Similarly, cultural traditions such as communal singing, storytelling, or dance can be incorporated into wellness programmes. These practices strengthen social bonds and mental well-being while respecting indigenous knowledge. By designing health "from home" and from community heritage, co-design fosters sustainable, culturally attuned care.

An example of institutional co-design is the Nityanand Integrated Medicine (NIMA) model in

Ajara, Maharashtra. Before starting NIMA, the founders had the opportunity to work in a government setup for handling the COVID-19 pandemic. Converting existing spaces during the pandemic—such as transforming a government hostel dining hall into a 50-bed COVID ICU with open windows—demonstrated this philosophy on an infrastructure level. The hall's natural ventilation, combined with family members providing nursing support (wearing masks, hand sanitiser, and learning simple breathing exercises for patients), created a supportive environment. Daily home-prepared herbal teas (*kashaya*) and simple homeopathic remedies were used alongside standard treatments. Clinicians observed that, in the second COVID wave, patients often needed oxygen support for shorter periods and steroid doses could be tapered more quickly than in the first wave. Although no randomised trial was performed, these observations gave confidence that supportive traditional measures, when used in concert with modern protocols, could improve outcomes.

Founded after the COVID-19 pandemic, NIMA houses modern medical and Ayurvedic services under one roof. In this setting, symptoms are treated promptly with allopathic medicine while Ayurvedic therapies address the root causes (*shodhana*). For instance, when a patient requires both hospitalisation and traditional cleansing therapies, the team coordinates their care integratively.

Illustrative Case Examples

Two patient cases from rural practice highlight how this integrative approach works in practice. The first case is of a middle-aged man with chronic psoriasis and psoriatic arthritis that had been managed for years with methotrexate and steroids. He had become steroid-dependent and could not stop it, even though he had severe gastritis. Integrative Ayurvedic therapies were introduced alongside his existing regimen. After three months, about 70 per cent of his skin lesions cleared. The steroid doses were gradually tapered off and then discontinued completely, and notably, the patient remained pain-free without them. Over time, his dermatological and joint inflammation became negligible, allowing clinicians to stop all immunosuppressant drugs. This outcome suggests that combining holistic Ayurvedic care with modern medicine can reduce reliance on aggressive drugs while effectively controlling autoimmune disease.

A second case involved a 22-year-old woman with a long history of chronic pancreatitis who contracted dengue fever, which led to viral hepatitis. During an acute pancreatitis flare, she experienced severe pain. The standard protocol was to transfer her to a tertiary care centre due to the dual organ involvement and high risk. The patient's family, however, chose to remain at the integrative rural centre. She was kept nil-by-mouth to rest the pancreas and given intravenous fluids. Since no oral medicines could be taken, an external Ayurvedic paste (*lepa*) was applied to her abdomen. Remarkably, she reported significant pain relief within six hours. Over the next two to three days, her food intake gradually resumed, and she recovered fully without needing an ICU transfer. This case illustrates how a carefully coordinated plan, resting the body with allopathic support while using traditional therapy externally, can complement standard care in an acute situation. It avoided the risks and costs of moving the patient far away, and the gentle, patient-centred approach (*saburi*) allowed healing to occur.

Discussion and Conclusions

These examples underline that integrative co-designed care can address both symptoms and underlying causes, often with fewer side effects. The organising principle of this model remains explicitly patient-centred: health systems and therapies are means to benefit the patient, not ends in themselves. No single medical tradition has all the answers. By combining the diagnostic precision and emergency care of modern medicine with the holistic, preventive wisdom of traditional practice, patients may receive the best of both worlds. However, implementation faces significant challenges. Some practitioners hold rigid views that only one system is valid, and legal or regulatory ambiguity can discourage integrated practice. To safeguard patients, clear documentation of each patient's history, treatments, and outcomes is essential. Such records ensure transparency and allow analysis of what works, turning anecdotal experience into shared knowledge. Communities should also be informed that traditional remedies can complement, but not replace, urgent medical interventions (informed consent is important), and that authorities should monitor any drug-herb interactions.

Despite these hurdles, global and national momentum supports integrative co-design. The World Health Organization's strategies and India's Ayush missions are building evidence and policy frameworks for blended care. Thousands of research studies are being collected in national portals to validate traditional therapies. Ultimately, the vision is that healthcare should serve people, not any single system. If each tradition's strengths are leveraged and its weaknesses minimised, then communities can receive more appropriate, comprehensive care. By rooting care in the home and culture, as well as in clinics, the "seeing with both eyes" approach creates a sustainable foundation for community wellness. Integrative medicine is not an end in itself but a practical response to the limits of fragmented care in rural India. Moving forward, it requires professional humility, interdisciplinary collaboration, and an unwavering focus on patients' needs. In this way, the best knowledge of modern science and traditional wisdom can work together to nurture the health of the whole community.

References

Donetto, S., Pierri, P., Tsianakas, V., & Robert, G. (2015). "Experience-based co-design and healthcare improvement: Realizing participatory design in the public sector". *The Design Journal*, 18(2), 227–248.

Ku, G. M. V. (2019). *Primary care for chronic conditions in rural India* [Doctoral dissertation, Maastricht University]. Maastricht University.

Kumar, R. (2024). "A family physician for all Indian families: A vision for 2047". *Journal of Family Medicine and Primary Care*, 13(10), 4125–4127.

Maslin-Prothero, S., Mastio, E., de Vries, K., & Galvin, K. T. (2023). "Co-design as enabling factor for patient-centred healthcare". *International Journal of Environmental Research and Public Health*, 20(10), 5782.

Pandey, P. & Sharma, S. (2017). "Is family medicine the answer to the shortage of specialist doctor in India?" *Journal of Family Medicine and Primary Care*, 6(2), 204–207.

Patwardhan, B. (2014). "Bridging Ayurveda with evidence-based scientific approaches in medicine". *EPMA Journal*, 5(1), 19.

https://doi.org/10.1186/1878-5085-5-19

Raina, S. & Navya. (2025). "An integrated approach in the present era: Scope and applications". *Journal of Ayurveda and Integrated Medical Sciences*, 10(1), 120–125.

Thakur, R., Jagota, A., & Thakur, S. (2024). "Personalized Ahara and Vihara: Aligning diet and lifestyle with Prakriti in Ayurveda for optimal health". *International Research Journal of Ayurveda & Yoga*, 7(11), 66–69.

Perspective 7

A Systems-Based Framework for Health Co-Design

R V Giridhar

CEO, Swami Dayananda Krupa Home

Kanchipuram

Introduction

Over the past two decades, health and design disciplines have increasingly converged around participatory, human-centred, and systems-oriented approaches. These developments reflect the growing recognition that health outcomes are shaped not only by medical interventions but also by environmental conditions, social relationships, behavioural patterns, and subjective experience. Global policy frameworks and national legislations emphasise dignity, inclusion, autonomy, and participation for individuals with physical, intellectual, and psychosocial disabilities.

Despite these advances, a persistent gap remains between conceptual intent and practical implementation. Many health systems continue to rely on linear, symptom-focused models that struggle to accommodate an individual whose cognitive, emotional, or behavioural profiles do not align with standard assumptions of autonomy, verbal communication, or decision-making capacity.

This gap is particularly evident in long-term residential care settings, where individuals require sustained support across multiple dimensions of functioning.

The paper addresses this gap by proposing a systems-based health co-design framework that reframes health as a dynamic process of alignment rather than a static state. Instead of positioning design as a technical solution to discrete problems, the framework conceptualises design as an ongoing process of shaping conditions that support regulation, participation, and well-being across time.

The framework is intentionally secular, interdisciplinary, and universally applicable. While informed by long-standing integrative perspectives on health and human functioning, the language, constructs, and arguments are grounded in contemporary scientific discourse, allowing the model to be evaluated, adapted, and applied across diverse cultural and institutional settings.

Limitations of Static Health Definitions

Conventional definitions of health often describe it as a state of complete physical, mental, and social well-being. While conceptually inclusive, such definitions remain operationally limited. They imply a static endpoint rather than an adaptive process and provide insufficient guidance for designing systems that respond to fluctuation, vulnerability, and long-term dependency.

In practice, health is rarely experienced as a stable condition. Instead, it emerges from continuous physiological regulation, emotional adaptation, cognitive processing, and social interaction. For individuals with developmental disabilities, chronic mental health conditions, or age-related cognitive decline, health is best understood as the capacity to maintain relative equilibrium in the face of ongoing internal and external change.

Health as Dynamic Homeostasis

From a systems science perspective, health can be conceptualised as dynamic homeostasis—the ability of a living system to sustain functional balance through continuous feedback and adjustment. This perspective aligns with research in physiology, neuroscience, and behavioural science, which demonstrates that well-being depends on the coordination of multiple subsystems rather than the optimisation of isolated variables.

In this view, health is not the absence of disruption but the presence of adaptive capacity. Emotional stress, sensory overload, social conflict, or environmental unpredictability can destabilise this balance, particularly for individuals with heightened sensory sensitivity or reduced regulatory flexibility.

Multi-Layered Dimensions of Health

Health emerges across interrelated dimensions that can be observed, influenced, and, to varying degrees, measured, as illustrated in the table given below:

Dimension	Observable Indicators	Examples of Measurement
Physical regulation	Vital signs, biomarkers, energy levels	Heart rate, sleep patterns
Emotional regulation	Stress response, mood stability	Stress scales, anxiety indices
Cognitive engagement	Attention, learning, adaptability	Task persistence, response flexibility
Social participation	Connection, cooperation, trust	Interaction frequency, social mapping
Existential coherence	Sense of meaning, belonging	Narrative analysis, resilience measures

These dimensions are not hierarchical but interdependent. Disruption in one domain often cascades into others, reinforcing the need for integrated rather than compartmentalised design approaches.

Redefining Design beyond Artefacts

Traditional design methodologies often focus on the creation of discrete artefacts—tools, products, or spatial configurations—intended to solve predefined problems. While such approaches have yielded significant advances, they are insufficient for addressing complex health contexts characterised by uncertainty, variability, and long-term relational dynamics.

In health co-design, the object of design is not merely a physical environment or service pathway but an ecosystem of interactions. This includes spatial layout, sensory qualities, temporal rhythms, social norms, communication styles, and participatory processes.

Alignment as a Design Goal

Within a systems-based framework, the primary goal of design is alignment—the degree to which internal states (physiological, emotional, and cognitive) are supported by external conditions (environmental, social, and organisational). Misalignment manifests as stress, behavioural deregulations, withdrawal, or conflict.

Design interventions that improve alignment do not necessarily require technological complexity. Small changes in lighting, sound, and predictability of routine or relational presence can significantly influence regulatory capacity and emotional stability.

Measurable Effects of Environmental and Relational Design

Research in environmental psychology and neurophysiology demonstrates that environmental features, such as natural light, acoustics, spatial openness, and sensory predictability, directly affect stress hormones, autonomic nervous system regulation, and emotional response patterns.

Similarly, relational factors, such as tone of voice, pacing of interaction, consistency of caregivers, and perceived emotional safety, have measurable effects on physiological coherence, often assessed through indicators such as heart rate variability (HRV).

Regulation as the Core of Well-Being

Across contemporary psychology and neuroscience, well-being is increasingly understood through the lens of regulation rather than pathology. Emotional, behavioural, and cognitive stability depend on the capacity of the nervous system to regulate arousal, attention, and response to stimuli. Deregulation—manifesting as anxiety, aggression, withdrawal, or sensory overload—is not inherently pathological but often reflects a mismatch between internal capacity and external demands.

Individuals with developmental disabilities or chronic psychosocial conditions typically exhibit narrower regulatory bandwidths. This makes them particularly sensitive to environmental unpredictability, excessive sensory input, and inconsistent relational cues. Health co-design, therefore, must prioritise regulatory support as a foundational objective.

Coherence and Psychophysiological Integration

Psychophysiological research highlights coherence—the synchronisation of heart rate, respiration, and emotional state—as a measurable indicator of well-being. High coherence states are associated with emotional stability, improved attention, and adaptive behaviour, while low coherence correlates with stress, impulsivity, and fatigue.

Design elements that promote coherence include:

- Predictable routines
- Sensory moderation
- Calm interpersonal pacing
- Meaningful engagement

These findings support the premise that health-supportive environments function as external regulators, particularly for individuals with limited internal self-regulation.

The Mind as a Distributed System

Rather than treating the mind as a single cognitive organ, contemporary psychology increasingly recognises it as a distributed system involving attention, memory, emotional processing, self-referential awareness, and social cognition. In practice, this means that health design must account for multiple psychological functions simultaneously.

For example:

- Excessive cognitive demand increases emotional reactivity.
- Emotional insecurity impairs learning and memory.
- Social exclusion exacerbates physiological stress responses.

A co-design approach that isolates one domain (e.g., medication compliance or task performance) without addressing others is unlikely to produce sustainable outcomes.

Health Design as an Experiential Process: Beyond Clinical Intervention

Health design is often equated with clinical intervention—diagnosis, treatment, and monitoring. However, lived health experience is shaped just as strongly by non-clinical variables, including space, rhythm, relationships, and participation.

From an experiential perspective, health is continuously "designed" through:

- How a space feels
- How time is structured
- How interactions unfold
- How individuals are invited to participate

Health co-design, therefore, involves intentional shaping of experience, not merely service delivery.

Story as Data: Narrative Indicators of Health

While quantitative measures remain essential, narrative observation provides critical insight into health dynamics, especially where verbal communication is limited. Behavioural shifts, emotional expressions, and changes in engagement patterns often precede measurable clinical change.

In residential care contexts, stories are not anecdotal embellishments but qualitative indicators of system alignment or misalignment. They reveal how design decisions interact with individual perception and regulation.

Practice-Based Observations from a Residential Care Organisation

The following cases are drawn from sustained observation within a long-term residential care organisation supporting adult men with developmental and psychosocial disabilities. The organisation functions as a closed ecosystem where environmental, relational, and routine-based variables can be systematically adjusted and observed over time.

These narratives are presented not as exceptional successes but as illustrative instances demonstrating how design-level interventions influence psychological and physiological outcomes.

Case Narrative 1: Sensory Environment and Anxiety Regulation

One resident exhibited pronounced anxiety during early evening hours, characterised by pacing, vocal distress, and agitation. Initial assessments focused on behavioural triggers and medication adjustment. However, longitudinal observation revealed a consistent environmental pattern: the resident's routine required passing through a narrow corridor with low lighting and high acoustic echo during the transition to evening rest.

Rather than escalating pharmacological intervention, the design team implemented environmental modifications. These included:

- Increased ambient lighting with softer tonal quality
- Acoustic dampening to reduce echo
- Introduction of a consistent evening ritual involving a low-effort, repetitive action performed at the same location daily

Within one week, observable anxiety behaviours reduced significantly. Over subsequent weeks, the resident began voluntarily initiating the evening transition with minimal prompting.

Interpretation

The intervention reduced sensory unpredictability and introduced rhythmic continuity, supporting autonomic regulation. The improvement illustrates how **environmental coherence can substitute for behavioural control**.

Case Narrative 2: Participatory Design and Spatial Meaning

During the redesign of an outdoor leisure area, one non-verbal resident repeatedly traced circular patterns on the ground while observing the construction site. Rather than redirecting the behaviour, the staff interpreted it as a form of spatial expression.

The final layout incorporated a circular pathway and seating arrangement. Post-construction observations indicated that the resident:

Spent increased time in the spaceDisplayed reduced agitation

Demonstrated greater tolerance for social proximity

Interpretation

This case demonstrates the value of **non-verbal participation** in co-design. When environments reflect individual expression, they foster familiarity, ownership, and emotional safety.

Case Narrative 3: Temporal Rhythm and Behavioural Stability

A period of increased behavioural deregulations across multiple residents coincided with irregular morning routines caused by staffing fluctuations. In response, the organisation introduced a simple, standardised morning structure. This included:

- Gentle physical movement at the same time daily
- Consistent auditory cues marking transitions
- Collective start to the day in a shared space
- Within two months, the staff reported:
- Improved attention during daytime activities
- Reduced interpersonal conflict
- Decreased need for behavioural intervention

Interpretation

Regular temporal rhythm functions as an **external organising principle**, particularly for individuals with limited internal time regulation.

Beyond Symptom Reduction: Measurement and Evaluation

Evaluating health co-design interventions requires moving beyond symptom reduction alone. Relevant indicators include:

- Frequency and intensity of deregulations episodes
- Duration of calm or engaged states
- Voluntary participation in activities
- Quality of social interaction
- Reduced reliance on coercive or restrictive practices

While not all outcomes lend themselves to standardised measurement, mixed-method approaches combining quantitative data with structured observation offer a robust evaluation strategy.

Relational Metrics

Relational stability—consistency of caregivers, predictability of interaction styles, and perceived emotional safety—emerges as a key mediator of health outcomes. Although difficult to quantify directly, relational variables can be indirectly assessed through:

- Staff turnover rates
- Incident reports
- Time-to-regulation following distress
- Resident-initiated interaction frequency

An Integrated Framework for Health Co-Design

Health co-design in complex care environments requires a structured yet flexible framework capable of addressing biological, psychological, social, and experiential dimensions simultaneously. Based on sustained observation and interdisciplinary synthesis, this paper proposes a multi-pillar framework that translates abstract systems principles into actionable design logic.

The framework does not prescribe uniform solutions; instead, it provides design orientations that can be adapted across contexts, populations, and resource settings.

Multi-Dimensional Integration for Systems-Based Health Co-Design

Health emerges from the interaction of multiple functional layers rather than isolated variables. Effective design interventions acknowledge this interdependence and avoid siloed solutions, as illustrated in the table below:

Design decisions that address only one layer often produce short-term gains but long-term instability. Integrated approaches support sustained regulation and engagement.

Design Focus	Description	Design Implication
Physical regulation	Bodily comfort and sensory moderation	Ergonomic layouts, sensory zoning
Emotional regulation	Safety, predictability, affect modulation	Consistent routines, calm interaction
Cognitive engagement	Attention, learning, adaptability	Task scaffolding, flexible pacing
Social participation	Belonging and cooperation	Shared spaces, group rituals
Existential coherence	Meaning and identity	Creative expression, contribution

Behavioural Patterning and Conditioning

Human behaviour is shaped not only by conscious choice but also by accumulated conditioning—habits, expectations, and learned responses. Health co-design must, therefore, engage with behavioural patterning, particularly in environments where individuals have limited capacity for verbal reasoning or abstract planning.

Design strategies include:

- Structuring environments to cue adaptive behaviour
- Reducing exposure to known stress triggers
- Reinforcing positive engagement through predictability rather than reward-punishment cycles

This approach aligns with contemporary behavioural science while avoiding coercive control mechanisms.

Empathic Regulation as Design Infrastructure

Empathy in care settings is often treated as an individual trait rather than a systemic property. In practice, empathic regulation must be designed into organisational systems.

Key elements include:

- Training the staff in non-reactive presence
- Establishing shared interaction norms
- Allowing time for relational pacing
- Designing spaces that reduce sensory and emotional overload for both residents and caregivers

When empathy is structurally supported, it reduces burnout among caregivers and improves stability among residents.

Role Alignment and Functional Clarity

Confusion of roles—among staff, residents, families, or administrators—introduces stress and conflict into care systems. Health co-design emphasises role clarity, ensuring that expectations are realistic, communicated, and aligned with capacity.

For residents, role alignment may involve:

- Assigning responsibilities based on interest and ability

- Offering consistent identity markers (e.g., "helper", "organiser", "caretaker")
- Avoiding infantilisation or unrealistic independence demands

Role clarity supports dignity and reduces anxiety arising from ambiguity.

Equilibrium and Inclusion

Equity in health design does not imply uniform treatment but balanced accommodation. Individuals require different forms of support to achieve comparable levels of participation and well-being.

Inclusive design, therefore, prioritises:

- Flexibility over standardisation
- Adjustment over normalisation
- Participation over performance

This orientation ensures that inclusion is operational rather than symbolic.

Co-Design beyond Verbal Input

Participation is often defined in terms of verbal feedback or explicit choice. In residential care contexts, this definition excludes individuals with limited speech or abstract reasoning ability.

A systems-based approach recognises non-verbal participation as equally valid. Indicators of participation include:

- Body orientation
- Repetition of action

- Emotional response
- Approach–avoidance patterns

Design processes that attend to these signals enable genuine inclusion without forcing verbal articulation.

Case Narrative 4: Relational Presence and De-escalation

One resident exhibited frequent emotional outbursts during evening hours, often leading to isolation as a risk management response. Rather than increasing behavioural control, caregivers experimented with quiet relational presence—remaining physically nearby without verbal instruction or demand.

Over time, the resident began to:

- Reduce intensity of distress behaviours
- Seek proximity rather than isolation
- Initiate shared activity

Interpretation

Relational presence functioned as a regulatory scaffold, illustrating that participation does not always require instruction or dialogue.

Health as a Collective Property

In closed or semi-closed residential systems, individual well-being is inseparable from collective dynamics. Emotional contagion, routine disruption, or staff stress can propagate quickly, affecting multiple residents simultaneously.

Health co-design, therefore, treats community structure itself as infrastructure, requiring intentional design.

- Key design elements include:
- Shared daily rituals
- Predictable communal transitions
- Opportunities for informal interaction
- Clear conflict de-escalation pathways

Shared Activity and Social Regulation

Group activities function as social regulators, synchronising attention, emotion, and movement. Simple shared actions, such as walking, stretching, listening to music, or meal preparation, create coherence that individual interventions often cannot.

These activities do not require therapeutic framing to be effective; their impact emerges from rhythm, repetition, and shared presence.

Rethinking Work in Care Settings

Work is often framed narrowly as productivity or skill acquisition. In health co-design, work is reconceptualised as purposeful engagement—activity that provides structure, identity, and contribution.

For individuals with developmental or psychosocial disabilities, meaningful engagement:

- Enhances self-regulation
- Reduces passive dependency
- Strengthens social identity

Capacity-Based Engagement Design

Rather than assigning tasks based on institutional need alone, engagement is designed around observed inclination and tolerance.

Examples include:

- Repetitive sorting or organising for individuals drawn to structure
- Rhythm-based activities for those responsive to movement or sound
- Care-related tasks for individuals oriented toward nurturing behaviours

Such alignment reduces resistance and increases voluntary participation.

Case Narrative 5 : Transforming Repetitive Behaviour into Contribution

One resident demonstrated persistent repetitive tapping behaviour. Instead of suppressing the action, the staff redirected it into structured rhythmic activity, integrating it into group-based engagement.

Over time:

- The behaviour became contextually appropriate
- The resident's social acceptance increased
- The resident's engagement duration extended without distress

Interpretation

Behaviours often labelled as "problematic" may represent misaligned capacity rather than dysfunction. Design reframing can transform such behaviours into assets.

Health Organisations as Adaptive Systems

Organisations delivering long-term care function as complex adaptive systems. Outcomes emerge not only from individual competence but also from interaction patterns among people, policies, spaces, and routines.

Health co-design, therefore, extends beyond resident-facing interventions to include:

- Staff workflow design
- Decision-making structures
- Feedback mechanisms
- Learning loops

Interdisciplinary Contribution

Designing for complex health contexts benefits from interdisciplinary collaboration. Inputs from psychology, architecture, engineering, occupational therapy, and design research enrich system adaptability.

However, interdisciplinary work must be coordinated through shared values of safety, dignity, and participation rather than discipline-specific dominance.

Advanced Concepts in Systems-Based Health Design

As health co-design frameworks mature, they must address not only functional outcomes but also subtler determinants of regulation, meaning, and sustainability. This section articulates advanced concepts that extend the framework beyond conventional clinical or design paradigms while remaining grounded in observable, research-aligned principles.

Design as a Participatory System Process

Health systems are often structured around hierarchical expertise, where decisions flow from professionals to recipients. Systems-based co-design reframes this structure by recognising that **participation itself alters system behaviour**.

Participation, in this context, is not limited to formal decision-making. It includes:

- Being consistently informed
- Being predictably included in routines
- Having one's responses shape environmental adaptation

When individuals experience participation—whether verbal or non-verbal—the system becomes more responsive, and resistance decreases. This aligns with research in organisational psychology demonstrating that perceived agency improves emotional regulation even in constrained environments.

Environmental Integration and Ecological Regulation

Environmental conditions exert continuous influence on physiological and psychological states. Health design that neglects environmental integration risks undermining even well-structured therapeutic programmes.

Key environmental variables include:

- Light (intensity, consistency, natural exposure)
- Sound (volume, predictability, resonance)

- Airflow and temperature
- Material texture and spatial proportion
- Visual openness versus enclosure

Studies in environmental psychology and biophilic design demonstrate that environments aligned with human sensory tolerance improve attention, reduce stress markers, and support emotional stability. In long-term care settings, these effects accumulate over time, producing measurable behavioural change.

Rhythm, Silence, and Cognitive Load

Modern care environments often emphasise activity and stimulation. However, excessive stimulation increases cognitive load, particularly for individuals with sensory sensitivity or limited attentional capacity.

Silence, understood scientifically as reduction of non-essential sensory input, plays a regulatory role by:

- Allowing autonomic down regulation
- Supporting memory consolidation
- Reducing emotional reactivity

Designing for silence does not imply inactivity. Instead, it involves intentional pacing, pauses between transitions, and spaces where sensory input is minimal and predictable.

From Accessibility to Experiential Inclusion

Accessibility is frequently defined through compliance with physical or procedural standards.

While necessary, this approach does not guarantee experiential inclusion.

Experiential inclusion focuses on:

- Whether individuals feel oriented rather than confused
- Whether spaces invite participation rather than avoidance
- Whether routines support competence rather than dependency

Inclusive design, in this sense, is not a static checklist but an ongoing adaptive process responsive to observed experience.

Design for Reduction of Suffering and Enhancement of Function

Health systems ultimately aim to reduce suffering and enhance functional participation. Systems-based co-design reframes this objective by emphasising **capacity restoration** rather than symptom elimination alone.

Key indicators of reduced suffering include:

- Shorter recovery time following distress
- Increased tolerance for uncertainty
- Improved social engagement
- Decreased need for restrictive or coercive practices

Importantly, success is not measured by conformity to normative behaviour but by relative improvement within individual capacity.

Ethical Neutrality and Scientific Universality

This framework is intentionally non-prescriptive and ethically neutral. It does not assume a particular cultural, philosophical, or belief system. Instead, it draws upon:

- Systems science
- Neurophysiology
- Environmental psychology
- Behavioural design
- Disability studies

By focusing on observable processes—regulation, coherence, participation, and alignment—the framework remains applicable across cultural contexts and institutional settings. Ethical considerations emerge from functional outcomes rather than normative ideology.

Implications for Policy, Design, and Research

Policymakers should consider shifting evaluation metrics from output-based compliance to process-based adaptability, particularly in long-term care environments.

Policy frameworks can support this shift by:

- Encouraging environmental and relational interventions
- Allowing flexibility in routine structuring
- Recognising qualitative indicators of well-being

Design Practice Implications

Design practitioners working in health contexts should expand their scope beyond spatial or product design to include:

- Temporal design (routines, transitions)
- Interaction design (communication patterns)
- Organisational design (roles, feedback loops)

Health co-design requires iterative observation and adjustment rather than one-time implementation.

Research Directions

Future research may explore:

- Longitudinal effects of environmental coherence
- Mixed-method measurement models combining physiological and narrative data
- Comparative studies across cultural and institutional contexts
- System-level predictors of caregiver sustainability and resident stability

Conclusions

This paper has presented a comprehensive systems-based framework for health co-design that integrates biological regulation, psychological experience, environmental context, and participatory process. By retaining complexity rather than simplifying it, the framework addresses populations and settings often marginalised by conventional health models.

The case narratives demonstrate that meaningful health improvement can emerge from modest, context-sensitive design interventions when systems are aligned to human regulatory capacity.

Health is not a static state to be achieved but a dynamic process to be supported. Design, when understood as system alignment rather than artefact creation, becomes a powerful tool for sustaining regulation, participation, and well-being.

A systems-based health co-design approach offers a scientifically grounded, universally applicable pathway for reimagining health environments, particularly those serving individuals with complex, long-term support needs. By focusing on alignment, adaptability, and experiential inclusion, such systems can reduce suffering while enhancing functional participation across diverse contexts.

Perspective 8

Skills Training for Public Health Education and Prevention of Noncommunicable Diseases

Dr Onkar Mittal
Swasth Hind, New Delhi

Background and Context

Effective primary health care involves promoting positive health attitudes, providing counselling on personal and family issues, offering nutrition and lifestyle guidance (including exercise), and ensuring early detection of priority diseases along with prompt primary treatment. Everyone should have access to a basic medical examination by a qualified provider and to essential tests (e.g., blood pressure, haemoglobin, blood sugar). Health education should teach simple preventive measures, such as 20 minutes of daily exercise that includes stretching, breathing techniques, and muscle-strengthening activities. Common complaints, such as chronic stress, should be investigated and addressed. Health education should accompany affordable care by explaining disease causes, treatment reasons, and the importance of adherence for chronic conditions such as hypertension, diabetes, anaemia, and joint pain.

Communities should keep a supply of essential medications so routine ailments can be treated locally. Residents generally respond well to advice on healthy living and adherence, indicating that community-based education can be effective. Local health educators can extend primary care into households. For example, trained village health educators can conduct house visits and health talks, reinforcing prevention messages. These educators would also facilitate referrals for specialised conditions (such as skin disorders, uterine prolapse, psychiatric illnesses, congenital heart disease, vision or dental issues) requiring clinic or hospital care. In this model, village health animators act as community-based educators. They conduct household visits and provide health education during weekly clinics, school programmes, and other community events. They keep records of individuals with chronic illnesses (e.g., hypertension, diabetes, anaemia) to ensure continuity of care and promotion of treatment adherence. They also gather community contributions for a village health fund.

At the ward level, health animators organise group meetings for families and older adults, conduct family health surveys, and maintain health service records.

They oversee a community drug chest and coordinate periodic medical examinations by qualified doctors for all households. By teaching basic exercises (stretching, breathing, muscle-strengthening) and healthy lifestyle practices, and by working with village health committees and health centres, health animators connect the community with the formal health system. In summary, these community educators expand preventive care and ensure primary care services (including referrals and campaigns) reach every village.

Training Needs and Model

Training village-level workers is a key innovation in current health initiatives. Existing frontline workers (ASHA and anganwadi workers) mainly focus on maternal and child health, leaving a gap in care for chronic diseases and older adults. To fill this gap, the proposed programme creates a role for health animators dedicated to noncommunicable diseases and elder care. Each health animator will complement existing workers by focusing on lifestyle-related illnesses among adults (especially those aged 45–70). The programme envisions each ward having one health animator who manages a community health fund (built from contributions and nominal user fees) to finance local primary care. Regular visits by NGO doctors or community health providers are arranged to support these activities and provide clinical oversight. In this way, structured training is introduced for prevention and early detection of chronic disease—training that is currently lacking in villages. The new training thus addresses a critical need by equipping local workers to lead grassroots health education, screening, and patient support.

Implementation Framework

The implementation plan establishes multiple levels of community health infrastructure. In each village, bi-monthly primary care clinics are organised (often led by visiting doctors) to provide regular access to medical services. Village health committees are formed to guide local health initiatives, supported by a ward-based community health fund. Each ward hosts a trained health animator who acts as the fund's coordinator. A village-level pharmacy (community drug chest) stocked with essential medicines is maintained to ensure treatment availability. Health animators and committee members receive training not only in health topics but also in the management and governance of community health activities. The village programme is linked with higher-level health services—clear referral pathways to nearby primary and community health centres are established, and experiences and data are shared with district and national health missions to align efforts. Community participation is central. An initial participatory needs assessment is conducted to inform programme design: households report recent out-of-pocket health expenditures and willingness to contribute financially to local care. These discussions help set realistic contribution levels for the community health fund and ensure support for the poorest.

Based on survey results, targets are set for household contributions to primary care and to a solidarity fund for people in need. The community's input directly shapes the scale of the health fund, the drug supply, and the services offered at each village and district level. A pilot project tests this framework in practice. In pilot wards, the whole package is deployed—a ward-level health office, a community drug chest, and a village health fund are established. Health animators and committees run regular clinics and outreach activities under the guidance of an NGO medical team. Linkages are maintained with government health centres for referral and supply of medicines. Lessons from the pilot are shared with district health authorities and national programmes. The pilot evaluates the feasibility of training health animators and refines training modules and operational processes. Its success could pave the way for scaling up the model while ensuring integration with existing health systems.

Conclusions

Fieldwork reveals a high prevalence of risk factors for chronic diseases among adults, especially those aged 45–70. These findings highlight the urgent need to act at individual, community, and system levels to prevent disease. The proposed certification programme offers an integrated framework that focuses on public health education, early diagnosis, and the management of chronic conditions through positive health promotion, nutrition advice, lifestyle counselling, and affordable primary care. Its core components are community-based—trained village health animators, active ward-level health committees, community drug stocks, health financing schemes, and regular outreach clinics. By empowering local health workers with targeted training in risk-factor prevention and patient education, the programme seeks to reduce the burden of noncommunicable diseases among older adults. Such coordinated efforts, aligned with national health strategies, are vital to enhancing population well-being and resilience in rural areas communities.

References

Chakma, J. K. & Gupta, S. (2014). "Lifestyle and non-communicable diseases: A double-edged sword for future India". *Indian Journal of Community Health,* 26(4), 325–332.

International Institute for Population Sciences (IIPS) & ICF. (2021). *National Family Health Survey (NFHS-5), 2019–21: India.* IIPS.

Jeet, G., Thakur, J. S., Prinja, S., & Singh, M. (2017). "Community health workers for non-communicable diseases prevention and control in developing countries: Evidence and implications". *PLoS ONE,* 12(7), e0180640.

Ministry of Health and Family Welfare, Government

of India. (2010). *National Programme for Prevention and Control of Cancer, Diabetes, Cardiovascular Diseases and Stroke (NPCDCS): Operational guidelines.*

Ramamoorthy, T., Leburu, S., Kulothungan, V., & Mathur, P. (2022). "Regional estimates of noncommunicable diseases associated risk factors among adults in India: Results from the National Noncommunicable Disease Monitoring Survey". *BMC Public Health*, 22, 1069.

Sharma, M., Gaidhane, A., & Choudhari, S. G. (2024). "A comprehensive review on trends and patterns of non-communicable disease risk factors in India". *Cureus*, 16(3), e57027.

World Health Organization. (2013). *Global action plan for the prevention and control of noncommunicable diseases 2013–2030.*

Perspective 9

Health Co-Design: Music as a Medium of Health

Arvindd Narayanan
Pratyusha Foundation, New Delhi

Introduction

Music occupies a unique position in the human experience, both as an art form and as a profound biological phenomenon. Across civilisations, music has been employed for ritual, healing, and self-expression. Shakespeare's observation, "If music be the food of love, play on," underscores an intuitive truth: music nourishes the emotional and spiritual dimensions of life.

In recent decades, empirical research has validated what ancient traditions long understood—sound and rhythm have measurable effects on the brain, body, and behaviour. Music therapy has now become an interdisciplinary field drawing from neuroscience, psychology, and ethnomusicology. It is increasingly recognised as a non-pharmacological intervention for a range of mental and physical disorders, integrating seamlessly with medical and spiritual models of health.

The Neuroscience of Music and Health

Listening to or producing music engages widespread neural circuits across both hemispheres of the brain. Functional MRI studies have shown activation in the auditory cortex, cerebellum, motor regions, limbic structures, and the prefrontal cortex. These areas coordinate sensory processing, emotion, attention, and motor control, explaining why music can simultaneously evoke movement, memory, and affective states.

The release of neurotransmitters such as dopamine, serotonin, and endorphins mediates the pleasure associated with music. Rhythmic patterns engage the basal ganglia, while melodic expectation activates reward networks in the ventral striatum, producing a sense of anticipation and resolution.

Physiological and Hormonal Effects

Music directly influences the autonomic nervous system. Studies indicate reductions in heart rate, blood pressure, and cortisol levels when individuals are exposed to calming or slow-tempo music. Conversely, stimulating music can enhance alertness and energy through increased sympathetic arousal.

Beyond relaxation, music modulates immune function. Group singing and chanting have been shown to elevate levels of immunoglobulin A, indicating improved immune response. Music also affects hormonal pathways by reducing cortisol and enhancing oxytocin, the "bonding hormone", thereby improving social connectedness and empathy.

Rhythm, Entrainment, and Neural Synchrony

A distinctive aspect of music's influence is neural entrainment—the synchronisation of brainwave frequencies with rhythmic external stimuli. Steady beats can align neural oscillations in the theta and alpha ranges, promoting focus and relaxation. This phenomenon underlies therapeutic applications in stroke and Parkinson's disease rehabilitation, where rhythmic auditory cues help restore motor coordination and gait regularity (Thaut et al., 2019).

Emotional and Psychological Dimensions of Music

Music serves as an external regulator of emotion, providing both catharsis and modulation. Research from McGill University suggests that listening to personally meaningful music activates brain regions linked to reward and emotional regulation. Patients with depression, anxiety, and PTSD often report significant reductions in symptom intensity following structured music therapy sessions.

The process mirrors cognitive behavioural therapy in that it allows individuals to reframe internal states through sound and expression. Music provides a safe space to articulate feelings that may be inaccessible through language, particularly in trauma and grief contexts.

Memory, Identity, and Healing

The mnemonic power of music is well-documented. In patients with Alzheimer's disease and dementia, exposure to familiar tunes often triggers autobiographical recall and emotional recognition. This link between sound and identity reaffirms the view that music sustains continuity of self even amidst cognitive decline.

Music's ability to activate the hippocampus and amygdala underlies these effects. Familiar melodies act as emotional cues, bridging the gap between memory and present awareness, a phenomenon increasingly harnessed in geriatric and palliative care.

Historical and Cultural Perspectives

From ancient Egypt to China, music has been interwoven with medicine. The Egyptians used chants in surgical rituals, while the Greeks believed in "musical ethos", the moral and physiological influence of modes. Pythagoras proposed that numerical ratios governing musical intervals also structured the cosmos, giving rise to the concept of *musica universalis*.

In Traditional Chinese Medicine, the five tones corresponded to the five elements and internal organs, each promoting specific emotional balance. Indigenous cultures across Africa and the Americas utilised drumming and collective song for communal healing and trance induction.

Indian Philosophy: *Nada Brahma* and *Raga Chikitsa*

In India, sound (*nada*) is conceived as the origin of creation, encapsulated in the phrase *Nada Brahma,* meaning, "the universe is sound." The *Sama Veda* and *Gandharva Veda* describe the therapeutic and ritual use of music, giving rise to *Raga Chikitsa,* the science of healing through melodic structures.

Texts such as the *Sangita Ratnakara* classify *ragas* not only by scale and emotion (*rasa*) but also by their effects on the mind and body. Each raga represents a vibrational field capable of influencing mood, energy, and physiology. The integration of sound and spirituality in Indian music underscores a holistic model where health is defined as *samatva*—equilibrium between the body, mind, and spirit.

Indian Classical Music and Healing

Empirical studies in India have validated ancient claims regarding the psychophysiological impact of ragas. For example:

- Raga Darbari Kanada has been shown to lower anxiety and blood pressure.
- Raga Bhairavi facilitates emotional catharsis and release of tension.
- Raga Desh refreshes the mood and stabilises cardiac rhythm.
- Raga Yaman/Kalyani enhances concentration and cognitive coherence.
- Raga Todi reduces hypertension and induces calm.

These effects are mediated through tempo, tonality, and emotional resonance, elements that mirror physiological rhythms such as heartbeat and breath.

Carnatic System: Precision and Breath as Therapy

In the Carnatic tradition, microtonal precision (*shruti*) and ornamental oscillations (*gamaka*) stimulate subtle neural pathways associated with emotion and attention. Singing requires sustained breath control, thereby enhancing vagal tone, improving respiratory efficiency, and promoting calm.

Compositions by saints such as Tyagaraja and Muthuswami Dikshitar exemplify *bhakti rasa*—devotional emotion that integrates lyrical meaning with structured melodic flow. The act of singing becomes a form of mindfulness, aligning intellect and emotion, leading to what psychologists describe as coherence between the heart and mind.

Chant, Rhythm, and Neural Coherence

Mantras and Vedic chants are another cornerstone of Indian sonic healing. The recitation of "AUM" aligns breathing patterns with parasympathetic dominance, reducing stress and enhancing clarity. Similarly, rhythmic cycles (*tala*) promote synchronisation across brain networks.

Drumming traditions, whether tribal, bhakti, or ritual, offer cathartic release and foster community bonding through collective rhythm. These practices mirror entrainment-based therapy, now used globally for trauma rehabilitation.

Comparative and Cross-Cultural Insights

Across civilisations, music functions as a medium of alignment—of the individual with self and the collective with community. Gregorian chants induce alpha wave dominance, signifying relaxed alertness, while African drum circles reinforce group cohesion through synchrony and empathy. Japanese koto and shakuhachi music exemplify simplicity and mindfulness, evoking calm through minimalism.

Despite diverse cultural forms, the underlying

mechanism remains consistent: structured sound entrains biological and emotional order, supporting mental equilibrium and resilience.

Modern Clinical and Social Applications

Contemporary hospitals employ music to reduce anxiety before surgery, alleviate pain during recovery, and improve mood in chronic illness. A 2018 meta-analysis in *The Lancet* confirmed that perioperative music significantly reduced pain perception and analgesic requirements (Bradt et al., 2018).

In neurology, Melodic Intonation Therapy (MIT) aids speech recovery in post-stroke aphasia, leveraging the brain's right-hemispheric melodic capacities (Schlaug et al., 2018). In psychiatry, structured listening and improvisation are used to manage depression, schizophrenia, and PTSD.

Music for Ageing and Dementia Care

Elderly care programmes integrating music report enhanced cognitive engagement and social interaction. The "Alive Inside" initiative, for example, demonstrated profound emotional awakening among dementia patients exposed to personalised playlists. Indian care institutions have begun experimenting with raga-based interventions in day-care and residential settings to address isolation and mood decline.

Everyday Wellness and Preventive Health

Beyond clinical settings, music contributes to preventive and lifestyle medicine. Examples include the following:

- Morning listening to energising ragas such as *Hamsadhwani* stimulates alertness.
- Afternoon instrumental music aids concentration.
- Evening ragas like *Darbari Kanada* or *Bageshree* induce relaxation and restorative sleep.

Mindful listening, i.e., treating sound as meditation, enhances emotional resilience and reduces fatigue, aligning with holistic wellness frameworks advocated by the World Health Organization (WHO, 2019).

Philosophical Integration: Science Meets Spirituality

Music bridges measurable neuroscience with intangible spirituality. On one hand, it regulates neural circuits, neurotransmitters, and hormones; on the other, it evokes transcendence and empathy. The Indian concept of Nada Brahma parallels modern physics' view of matter as vibration, suggesting that all existence is rhythmic.

Health, in this sense, becomes harmony, the resonance between physiological rhythm and universal sound. This synthesis embodies a bio-psycho-spiritual model where healing arises from coherence among the body, mind, and spirit.

As Hans Christian Andersen observed, "Where words fail, music speaks." The enduring universality of music lies in its capacity to unify emotion, cognition, and consciousness, transforming both individual and collective well-being.

Conclusions

Music is more than an art; it is a dynamic field of energy that interacts with biology and consciousness. From neural entrainment to spiritual awakening, it operates across the full spectrum of human experience. As modern science validates ancient insights, music therapy emerges as a bridge between disciplines—art and medicine, science and spirituality.

The convergence of empirical research and traditional wisdom affirms that sound, when consciously applied, can heal, harmonise, and humanise. In an increasingly fragmented world, music remains a universal language of restoration and connection, an accessible, evidence-based medium of health for the body, mind, and soul.

References

- Chanda, M. L. & Levitin, D. J. (2013). "The neurochemistry of music". *Trends in Cognitive Sciences, 17*(4), 179–193.
- Koelsch, S. (2014). "Brain correlates of music-evoked emotions". *Nature Reviews Neuroscience, 15*(3), 170–180.
- Kreutz, G., Bongard, S., Rohrmann, S., Grebe, D., Bastian, H. G., & Hodapp, V. (2004). "Effects of choir singing or listening on secretory

immunoglobulin A, cortisol, and emotional state". *Journal of Behavioral Medicine, 27*(6), 623–635.

- Nozaradan, S., Peretz, I., & Mouraux, A. (2012). "Selective neuronal entrainment to the beat and meter embedded in a musical rhythm". *Journal of Neuroscience, 32*(49), 17572–17581.
- Schlaug, G., Marchina, S., & Norton, A. (2010). "From singing to speaking: Facilitating recovery from nonfluent aphasia". *Annals of the New York Academy of Sciences, 1169*(1), 446–454.
- Thaut, M. H. & Hoemberg, V. (Eds.). (2014). *Handbook of Neurologic Music Therapy.* Oxford University Press.
- Thaut, M. H., McIntosh, G. C., & Hoemberg, V. (2015). "Neurobiological foundations of neurologic music therapy: Rhythmic entrainment and the motor system". *Frontiers in Psychology, 5,* 1185.
- World Health Organization. (2019). *Health Evidence Network synthesis report 67: What is the evidence on the role of the arts in improving health and well-being?* WHO Regional Office for Europe.
- Krishna, R., Sriram, S., & Ramakrishnan, S. (2022). "Evaluating Carnatic raga-based interventions on stress and mood: A pilot randomized controlled study". *Indian Journal of Psychological Medicine, 44*(5), 456–464.

Perspective 10

Health Co-Design: Dance as a Medium of Health

Riddhi Mehar
Anaadikruti, New Delhi

Introduction

Wellness in contemporary discourse is no longer confined to the absence of disease or the maintenance of physical fitness. It is increasingly understood as an integrated ecosystem encompassing emotional balance, cognitive clarity, social belonging, and subtle energetic alignment. Within this expanded framework, the Health Co-Design initiative sought to explore how culturally rooted knowledge systems may contribute meaningfully to holistic well-being. In this context, Indian classical music and dance emerge not merely as artistic traditions but as embodied, neurologically coherent, and culturally intelligent pathways to health.

Representing the dance perspective at the Health Co-Design Conference, this paper proposes that Indian classical dance functions as a living methodology of health. It is rooted in the dynamic interplay of body, mind, emotion, energy, and environment. While informed by broader cosmological and elemental philosophies, its central insight remains accessible and direct: dance organises human energy toward wholeness.

Dance as an Experiential Pathway to Holistic Health

Dance may be understood as a form of living medicine, an integrative practice in which physical movement, emotional expression, cognitive engagement, energetic awareness, and cultural memory converge. It is not merely a cultural artefact preserved for performance; rather, it is an embodied architecture of health and a lived science of alignment. Through disciplined movement and expressive intention, dance synchronises physiological processes with psychological states, enabling the practitioner to experience coherence across multiple dimensions of being.

Within Indian classical traditions such as Kathak, dance becomes a structured yet fluid methodology that integrates rhythm, gesture, narrative, and breath. It transforms movement into insight and expression into regulation, offering a systematic pathway toward internal harmony.

Philosophical Foundations: Dance as Energy in Motion

Indian aesthetic thought has long conceptualised movement as a dialogue between the individual and the cosmos. Every gesture, breath, and rhythmic articulation carries an energetic imprint. Dance thus operates as a bridge between the visible and the invisible—between physical form and subtle states of emotion and consciousness. It becomes a carrier (*vāhak*) of transformation, a process through which rhythm regulates the nervous system and movement becomes medicine.

In this philosophical orientation, dance is not a leisure activity or performance skill alone. It is a technology of awareness and identity formation. By engaging rhythm, breath, and intentional gesture, the practitioner recalibrates internal energy patterns, harmonising physiological states with emotional and cognitive processes. The body becomes both instrument and site of knowledge.

Synchronisation of Body, Breath, and Being

Contemporary wellness science emphasises coherence among bodily rhythms, respiration, and mental focus as foundational to health. Classical dance practices naturally cultivate this coherence. In Kathak, for instance, rhythmic precision, intricate footwork, expressive storytelling, and structured improvisation demand acute sensory awareness and breath regulation. Rhythm stabilises biological oscillations; expressive movement facilitates psychological release; and choreographic structure promotes neurological integration.

Through sustained practice, dancers develop heightened proprioceptive awareness, refined vestibular balance, and enhanced motor coordination. The repeated alignment of movement with rhythmic cycles induces regulatory effects on the autonomic nervous system, supporting stress modulation and emotional equilibrium. Dance thus becomes a practical system for achieving embodied presence.

Dance and Emotional Intelligence

As a narrative performing art, classical dance provides a dynamic framework for exploring archetypes, identities, and emotional states. The practitioner inhabits emotions such as love, longing, devotion, separation, conflict, and joy, not as abstract concepts but as lived, embodied experiences. This process creates a safe container for emotional exploration and catharsis.

By learning to experience intense emotions without being overwhelmed by them, dancers cultivate emotional resilience and empathic intelligence. They acquire the capacity to feel deeply while remaining centred. In this way, dance fosters psychological maturity: it refines emotional literacy while reinforcing internal stability.

Conscious Movement and Psychophysical Integration

Dance introduces the principle of intentional movement—movement that is mindful, rhythmically structured, breath-anchored, and expressively embodied. This form of movement differs fundamentally from routine or utilitarian motion. It activates motor cognition, strengthens cross-hemispheric coordination, enhances proprioceptive pathways, and engages emotional memory networks.

Through such integrated activation, dance elevates internal awareness. The body learns before the mind conceptualises; embodied experience precedes analytical understanding. This reversal of conventional learning hierarchies is itself therapeutic, restoring trust in somatic intelligence and reinforcing the unity of sensation, cognition, and insight.

The Tripartite Lens: Experiencing, Method, Understanding

Dance may be understood through a tripartite framework: experiencing (अनुभूति), method (पद्धति), and understanding (परिभाषा). First, the dancer undergoes direct, somatic experience; emotional intelligence becomes embodied intelligence. Second, disciplined technique provides methodological structure, creating a container within which creativity and clarity can emerge. Finally, the integration of experience and method yields insight. Knowledge is not externally imposed but internally realised.

This cyclical movement from sensation to structure to understanding mirrors processes of growth in life itself. It reinforces a pedagogy in which wisdom arises through lived engagement rather than abstraction alone.

Physiological, Cognitive, and Emotional Contributions to Wellness

From a physiological perspective, classical dance strengthens neuromuscular coordination and bilateral integration, aligning motor pathways across the body. Sustained rhythmic sequences build cardiovascular endurance and muscular strength, while disciplined posture and spinal alignment reduce long-term structural imbalances. Over time, practitioners develop refined kinaesthetic intelligence, becoming acutely aware of spatial orientation, balance, and directional shifts.

Psychologically, dance facilitates emotional regulation by enabling the release of embodied stress patterns. The rhythmic and expressive dimensions of practice stimulate parasympathetic activation, reducing the physiological markers of chronic stress. Simultaneously, choreographic learning enhances memory retention, sequential processing, attentional control, and executive functioning. Rhythm-based cognition improves neural synchronisation, fostering clarity and focus. Movement, in this sense, becomes a form of meditation—anchoring awareness in the present moment.

Energetic Alignment and Spiritual Integration

Beyond measurable physiological and cognitive effects, dance engages subtler dimensions of human experience. Through the integration of breath, gesture, and focused awareness, practitioners often report a sense of internal spaciousness and expanded perception. Classical dance traditions frame this as harmonisation of subtle energies, a unification of body, mind, and spirit.

In cultivating this integration, dance expands one's inner capacity (पात्रता) to perceive, feel, and transcend habitual patterns. It elevates consciousness not through abstraction but through embodied refinement. The practitioner develops a heightened sensitivity to inner and outer rhythms, fostering clarity, insight, and equilibrium.

Cultural Grounding and Identity Formation

Dance does not operate in isolation from culture. It situates the practitioner within lineage, tradition, mythology, music, and shared aesthetic codes. This cultural embedding provides psychological grounding and a sense of belonging. Identity becomes both fluid and anchored—capable of exploration yet supported by continuity.

Participation in classical dance communities also

fosters interpersonal sensitivity and collective resonance. Shared rhythm and narrative generate social cohesion, reinforcing emotional bonds and mutual empathy. Thus, dance contributes not only to individual well-being but also to communal harmony.

Dance as a Technology of Self-Elevation

When viewed holistically, dance may be described as a technology of self-elevation. It constructs an internal architecture composed of discipline, surrender, exploration, and insight. Within this structured yet expansive space, the practitioner can inhabit strength and vulnerability, fluidity and grounding, introspection and expression.

By integrating physical vitality, emotional literacy, cognitive precision, energetic awareness, and cultural continuity, dance becomes a comprehensive ecosystem of well-being. It is not an auxiliary wellness tool but a co-designer of health, an embodied system through which the individual reorganises the whole being.

Conclusions: Dance as Co-Designer of Holistic Health

Dance, therefore, transcends its conventional classification as performance art. It is an integrated methodology of human flourishing. Within the Health Co-Design framework, it becomes evident that dance offers a powerful entry point into holistic health—movement evolves into meditation, emotion into insight, rhythm into alignment, and the body into a doorway to inner coherence.

References

1. *The Natyasastra*. Manomohan Ghosh (Trans.). Calcutta: The Asiatic Society, 1961.
2. *Abhinaya Darpana*. Manomohan Ghosh (Trans.). Calcutta: Firma KLM Private Ltd., 1957
3. Vatsyayan, K. *Classical Indian Dance in Literature and the Arts*. New Delhi: Sangeet Natak Akademi, 1968.
4. Damasio, A. *The Feeling of What Happens*. New York: Harcourt Brace, 1999.
5. Kolk, Bessel van der. *The Body Keeps the Score*. New York: Viking (Penguin Group), 2014.
6. Fraleigh, S. H. *Dance and the Lived Body*. Pittsburgh: University of Pittsburgh Press, 1987.
7. Coomaraswamy, A. K. *The Dance of Shiva*. New York: The Sunwise Turn, 1918.

Perspective 11

Rethinking Health Policy in India: Why Community Co-Design Matters More Than Experiments

Guriqbal Singh

Civic Action Labs, New Delhi

Background

Health policy in India, and globally, is highly enamoured with experimental approaches, RCTs, pilots, and innovation labs. There's merit to evidence-based policymaking, obviously. But I'm worried that in the pursuance of scientific innovation, we have forgotten people and communities are not just subjects but also part of our pursuance toward more knowledge. We've gone too far in treating communities like laboratories where we test interventions designed elsewhere, completely aloof from the angle of participation. The metaphor itself is revealing. Laboratories are controlled spaces where variables are isolated and measured; communities aren't like that. Health isn't like that either, especially when you're talking about well-being that's tied up with social relationships, cultural practices, and ecological knowledge, all the messy stuff that experimental design tries to control. This style of intervention, with all due respect to the good intention and cause that it caters to, makes health synonymous with disease, problem, medicine, vaccination, etc., which itself is injustice to health and the vastness that it carries.

Looking at three cases—the Mitanin health worker programme in Chhattisgarh, mental health initiatives in North India, and traditional healing in the Himalayas—I argue for what I tentatively call "policy companionship". I know the term needs work, but bear with me. The basic idea is moving away from the notion of the state as an external experimenter toward the state as a genuine partner, not doing research on communities but with them. It's a shift that matters not only ethically but also practically. These cases show better outcomes when communities are treated as knowledge producers rather than test subjects.

The paper makes two claims. First, experimental governance has inherent limits, particularly when dealing with traditional medicine and folk healing systems. You can't extract these practices from their social context without fundamentally changing what they are. Second, co-design isn't just better methodology. It's an ethical requirement when you're working with knowledge systems that mainstream policy has historically marginalised or appropriated. The cases demonstrate what this looks like in practice and why it produces more sustainable, legitimate health governance.

The Problem with Laboratories

As the discussion and churnings on the importance and vitality of indigenous knowledge systems in cultures is taking the front seat in global thought, it made me think about the homogeneity of health interventions and their practices presented to the communities by way of imposition, where communities from different cultures, geographies, and regions perceive materials, nature, and healing uniquely. They carry their own belief systems with regard to health and healing, which we broadly call as "traditional methods". What struck me wasn't the disagreement about whether traditional methods work or not. That debate's been on for a long time. It was the unexamined assumption that the way to figure this out is through controlled trials and standardised protocols, as if the question is just technical rather than fundamentally about different ways of knowing.

Over the past 20 years, experimental approaches have basically taken over development policy. RCTs, pilots, and innovation labs are everywhere now, especially in the Global South. Deaton and Cartwright (2018) wrote a paper critiquing this turn, pointing out that even when RCTs are done well, there are still serious questions about external validity and causal inference. Just because something works in a controlled setting doesn't mean it'll work when you scale it up in reality. Peters et al. (2018) systematically reviewed RCTs in developing countries and found that most published studies don't even discuss hazards to external validity, like Hawthorne effects, general equilibrium effects, or special care in treatment provision. Pritchett and Sandefur (2015) go further, showing that applying rigorous evidence from one context to another can actually reduce predictive accuracy compared to using local evidence, even if that local evidence is biased.

But there's a deeper issue that Scott (1998) revealed in *Seeing Like a State*. The high-modernist state wants legibility. It wants to make society readable, measurable, and controllable. This impulse isn't inherently bad. Sometimes you need standardisation. But when you're dealing with health systems that are embedded in local culture, ecology, and social relationships, the drive to make everything legible ends up destroying the very things that make those systems work.

Here's what I mean. In rural India, people don't go to doctors or traditional healers based on what's medically effective, however you define that. They go based on trust, on who their neighbours consult, on spiritual beliefs, on what their grandmother told them, on whether the practitioner speaks their language and respects their customs. All of that is signal, not noise. However, experimental governance treats it as noise to be filtered out rather than knowledge to engage with.

This becomes especially problematic with traditional medicine. When policy tries to formalise and integrate practices like Ayurveda or folk healing, it almost always does so on biomedical terms, which means asking: Can we prove this works by our metrics? Can we standardise this into our system? The questions that should be asked instead are: What do communities already know that we should learn from? How can formal health systems support rather than replace what's already working? Lambert (2015) documents how formalisation processes valorise "epistemic" expertise over "performative" expertise acquired through experiential learning and oral traditions, effectively marginalising traditional practitioners.

So, policy companionship, and again, I'm open to better terms, means shifting from experiments on communities to knowledge creation with them—not short-term pilots but sustained relationships, not external expertise imposed from above but policymakers positioned as learners, not treating communities as test populations but as partners with valuable knowledge. The three cases from India mentioned earlier show what this looks like and why it matters.

Why Experimental Governance Falls Short: Limits of Controlled Trials

I'm not anti-RCT. Banerjee and Duflo did important work and deserve the accolades they received. The problem isn't randomised trials per se. It's when they become the only thing we trust, the only kind of evidence that counts. Deaton and Cartwright (2018) emphasise this point well. Even technically sound RCTs face serious issues with generalisability. If something is tested in one context under controlled conditions, it is assumed it'll work the same way everywhere else.

Indian health systems are complicated in ways that resist experimental isolation. Whether someone seeks healthcare depends on dozens of factors, such as trust in providers, gender dynamics, who decides if women can leave the house, what the neighbours will think, previous experiences, economic constraints, and spiritual beliefs about illness and healing. You can't control all these factors. More importantly, you shouldn't want to, because these factors aren't external variables; they're the actual context in which health happens.

Scott's (1998) critique is useful here. He argues that high-modernist planning fails when it tries to impose simple, legible order on complex local realities. The state wants to see clearly, which requires simplification. But simplification means loss. When you standardise health practices so they're legible to bureaucrats in Delhi, you lose the embedded knowledge that makes them work in specific communities. Traditional healing gets dismissed as superstition or, worse, gets appropriated and formalised in ways that strip it of social meaning.

Extraction vs. Genuine Partnership

There's a pattern I keep seeing in how mainstream health policy engages with traditional medicine. It goes something like this: Acknowledge that people use these practices. Study them to see if they work. Take the ones that do, by biomedical standards. Formalise them. Integrate them into the official system. This sounds reasonable, except that the communities and practitioners where this knowledge comes from rarely have meaningful say in the process. Their knowledge gets extracted, standardised, and institutionalised, but they're left out.

Mishra (2018) documents how rural communities continue consulting folk practitioners despite minimal government support. This is so not because they don't have access to biomedical care, though that's sometimes true, but because these practitioners offer something different. They're embedded in social relationships, share community cosmologies, and understand illness in holistic rather than purely physiological terms. When policy tries to replace or formalise these practices without understanding their social function, it usually fails. Or it succeeds on its own narrow terms—more certified practitioners, more AYUSH facilities—while actually dismantling the community infrastructure people depend on.

I call this epistemic extraction—taking knowledge from communities to validate externally-designed interventions without genuine partnership or recognition. This is visible in AYUSH mainstreaming efforts. Yes, there's more institutional integration now, but who designs the policies? Who decides what counts as legitimate practice? Who benefits when traditional knowledge gets formalised and monetised? This usually does not include the communities where it originated. Patwardhan et al. (2023) point out that epistemic injustice to traditional medicine knowledge has contributed to the benefits of AYUSH systems remaining unappreciated, even as research methods remain fixated on evidence from biomedical frameworks.

The alternative, what I call policy companionship, begins from a different premise. Communities aren't just sources of data or test sites for interventions. They're knowledge producers with valid expertise that might be fundamentally different from technical knowledge but no less valuable. Blomkamp (2018) argues that co-design is fundamentally about power and legitimacy. Real co-design challenges traditional hierarchies.

Case Study : What Partnership Actually Looks Like The Mitanin Programme in Chhattisgarh

The Mitanin programme offers probably the best example I know of policy companionship in Indian health governance. Launched in 2002, it trained community health workers, mostly women from marginalised communities, to provide basic healthcare and mobilise communities around social determinants of health.

What makes it different isn't just that it worked but how it worked.

From the beginning, the programme was designed with strong community participation. Nandi and Schneider (2014) document how Mitanins weren't just implementing health interventions designed elsewhere. They were identifying local health needs, mobilising communities, and addressing social determinants like water, sanitation, and domestic violence. The programme recognised that health workers' effectiveness depends on their embeddedness in community trust networks, not just technical training.

This matters because community health worker programmes often fail when workers are positioned as outsiders or mere implementers. Scott et al. (2019) show how ASHAs (Accredited Social Health Activists) in other states face serious challenges due to India's rigid hierarchical health system structure, work overload, and inadequate system support. The difference with Mitanin is structural. Workers have more autonomy, better support systems, and crucially, their local knowledge is valued rather than dismissed.

Recent research by Desai et al. (2024) on urban ASHAs in Punjab reveals systemic barriers, including unfilled supervisory positions, minimal collaboration with community engagement structures, and populations far exceeding guidelines. ASHAs are regularly assigned ad-hoc work without compensation, facing precarious working conditions due to their designation as volunteers rather than workers with labour rights.

This contrasts sharply with the Mitanin model, where community embeddedness and recognition of workers' knowledge are central design features.

The outcomes speak for themselves—better maternal health indicators, improved immunisation coverage, increased community mobilisation around health. But more importantly, the process created sustainable infrastructure. Communities weren't passive recipients. They were partners in designing and implementing health interventions relevant to their specific contexts.

Mental Health and Community Participation

Mental health work in North India offers another angle on why partnership matters. Mathias et al. (2022) studied community-based mental health services delivered through ASHAs and found something interesting. When health workers had strong community connections and were supported to engage in genuine dialogue rather than just implement protocols, mental health outcomes improved significantly.

The fact is that mental health is deeply tied to social context, cultural beliefs about illness, and community support networks. You can't just impose biomedical psychiatric protocols and expect them to work. Communities have their own understandings of mental distress, their own support systems, and their own healing practices. Effective mental health intervention has to engage with rather than replace these existing frameworks.

The successful programmes Mathias and his colleagues studied weren't extractive. They didn't just train health workers in Western psychiatric models and send them out. Instead, they created space for dialogue between different knowledge systems. Health workers learned to navigate between biomedical frameworks and community understandings, serving as bridges rather than replacements.

This required policymakers to position themselves differently, not as experts with answers but as partners in figuring out what mental health support looks like in specific communities. It meant accepting that their technical knowledge, while valuable, wasn't sufficient. Community knowledge about social relationships, cultural practices, and existing support systems was equally necessary.

Traditional Healing in Kinnaur

The most striking case, to me, is of the traditional therapeutic practices in Kinnaur, Himachal Pradesh. Sharma et al. (2025) conducted a qualitative study documenting how traditional healing there integrates herbal medicine, ritual practices, and ecological knowledge into a coherent system. It's not just about treating symptoms. It's a whole cosmology of health and well-being.

Here's what makes this relevant to policy. Government AYUSH integration efforts have largely failed to engage meaningfully with practices like these. The impulse is to formalise, standardise, and certify—extract the herbal remedies that can be proven effective by biomedical metrics, and dismiss the rest as superstition. But that completely misses the point. You can't separate herbal knowledge from the social and spiritual context. The efficacy, if we're going to use that word, comes from the whole system, not just the plants.

This is what I mean when I speak of epistemic extraction. When policy tries to make these practices legible to the state, it necessarily transforms them into something else. The state wants to know: Which herbs work? What are the dosages? What are the conditions? Can we standardise protocols? But traditional healing in places like Kinnaur isn't organised around these questions. It's organised around maintaining relationships between people, between communities and their environment, between the physical and spiritual dimensions of health.

Kudlu (2025) examines how India's technoscientific and economic imaginaries have converged in traditional medicine policy, bringing it into the fold of state science not through epistemic integration but as a regulatory object and export asset. The state positions itself as the arbiter of Ayurveda's global legitimacy through the language and apparatus of science, prioritising access to lucrative markets within policy. This creates fundamental tensions because scientisation is just one strategy among several, and it often conflicts with the experiential and relational nature of traditional healing.

Trying to validate these through biomedical trials

misses the point entirely. It's like asking whether prayer works by measuring biochemical outcomes. The wrong framework is being applied. Patwardhan et al. (2023) emphasise that an intervention that millions find safe and effective constitutes stronger evidence than small controlled studies, yet research methods remain fixated on particular study designs rather than evolving with the dynamism of actual practice.

Policy companionship here means asking different questions entirely—not can we prove these practices work by our standards, but how can formal health systems support what communities are already doing? How do we create governance frameworks that allow space for knowledge that resists standardisation? How do we learn from them rather than extract from them? These are tougher questions because they require humility about the limits of external expertise, but they're the right ones if you take seriously the idea that communities might know something you don't.

Co-Design as More than Methodology

Co-design is much discussed in policy circles these days, usually as a technique for better outcomes. However, Blomkamp (2018), and more recently, Mintrom and Einfield (2024) argue it's fundamentally about power and legitimacy. Who decides what counts as knowledge? Who sets priorities? Who has authority? As mentioned earlier, co-design challenges traditional hierarchies.

There's a big difference between genuine co-design

and what usually happens. Extractive consultation is where community input validates decisions already made. Real co-design means communities shape policy from conception, not just react to draft plans. It means recognising different kinds of expertise as equally valid. A traditional healer with 40 years of experience knows things a public health Ph.D. holder doesn't, and vice versa. The question is whether policy can hold both kinds of knowledge together without one colonising the other.

Mintrom and Einfield (2024) identify co-design as a participatory and design-oriented process that creatively and actively engages diverse participants to define and address public problems. Evidence suggests it's especially useful in broadening participation, encouraging creative speculation about future outcomes, and prototyping policy approaches. But the key is that it has to be genuine. Participants must have real power to shape outcomes, not just provide input that is filtered through predetermined frameworks.

Blomkamp's (2021) work on systemic design practice for participatory policymaking shows how government departments adopting systems thinking, human-centred design, and co-design principles reflect a broader participatory turn in public administration. The spread of public sector innovation labs contributes to the popularity of "designerly" methods emphasising empathy and creativity. But there are significant challenges to embedding these methods in organisations structured around hierarchy and technical expertise.

Policy companionship extends this by emphasising time and relationship. Not one-off consultations but ongoing engagement. Not short pilots with predetermined endpoints but open-ended partnerships. Not external experts who swoop in and leave but policymakers who position themselves as learners embedded in communities for the long haul. It's fundamentally different from experimental governance. It is less about control, more about collaboration and mutual transformation.

What Would This Actually Look Like? A Tentative Framework

Based on these cases and studying what they have in common, I propose four principles for policy companionship. These are provisional, as I'm still working through the implications.

1. **Shared authority over knowledge**
   Communities don't just get consulted. They help define what questions matter and what counts as valid knowledge. Traditional and experiential knowledge aren't inputs to a process; they're frameworks for understanding health that might be fundamentally different from biomedical approaches. The state needs to be receptive of this plurality. Patwardhan et al. (2023) emphasise the need to recognise local epistemic expertise, local forms of care, and the contributions communities make to overall population health.

This requires acknowledging that current health system models must evolve beyond biomedical dominance.

2. **Long-term relationships over interventions**
   Pilots have endpoints; companionship doesn't. The goal isn't to test and scale but to build ongoing capacity for mutual learning and adaptation. This is less efficient in the short term but probably more sustainable. Nandi and Schneider (2014) show how the Mitanin programme's long-term community embeddedness produces better outcomes than short-term intervention models.
3. **Recognition of plural knowledge systems**
   Not everything can or should be made legible to the state. Some practices work precisely because they're local, contextual, and resistant to standardisation. Policy needs to create space for that rather than trying to eliminate it in the name of efficiency or scalability. Sharma and his colleagues (2025) demonstrate how Kinnaur's traditional healing practices derive their efficacy from integration with social, ecological, and spiritual contexts that cannot be extracted without fundamentally altering the practice.
4. **Policymakers as learners**
   This requires real humility. It means acknowledging technical expertise has limits, being open to having core assumptions challenged, and accepting that communities might know better about their own needs. This

is uncomfortable for professionals trained to be experts. But it's necessary if you're serious about partnership rather than extraction. Mintrom and Luetjens (2016) note that design thinking in policymaking requires policymakers to adopt empathetic inquiry and iterative learning, positioning themselves as collaborators rather than experts with predetermined solutions.

None of this means abandoning evidence or rigour. It means understanding that rigour looks different when you're dealing with complex social systems rather than controlled experiments. It means evidence has to include community knowledge, oral histories, and traditional practices, not just data from external observers with clipboards.

Conclusion: Where This Leaves Us

So, where does this leave health policy in India? The experimental paradigm isn't going away. There's too much invested in it, too many careers built around it, and too many institutional incentives. But there's also growing recognition that it's insufficient, particularly for traditional medicine, mental health, anything where cultural context matters deeply.

The cases I've discussed suggest alternatives are possible. When the state positions itself as companion rather than experimenter, when communities are treated as knowledge producers rather than test subjects, outcomes improve. More importantly, the process becomes more just. That matters independently of measurable health outcomes.

This isn't just about effectiveness, though it is more effective. It's about legitimacy. In pluralistic societies like India, governance can't succeed by imposing uniformity. It has to work with difference, learn from it, build with it. Traditional healing systems aren't obstacles to modern healthcare. They're different ways of knowing and practising that can coexist with biomedical approaches if policy creates space for that coexistence. Kudlu (2025) notes that India's traditional medicine policy has entered a dynamic phase with rising budgets and curriculum reforms, but the emphasis on innovation and global market positioning risks further scientisation that may undermine the very qualities that make traditional medicine valuable to communities. The challenge is creating policy frameworks that support rather than extract from traditional knowledge systems.

The shift from laboratories to companionship is a big one. I'm under no illusions about how hard it would be institutionally. It requires rethinking what states do, how professionals are trained, what counts as successful policy, and how resources are allocated. It challenges many comfortable assumptions about expertise and evidence.

But the alternative, continuing to treat communities as laboratories, isn't working, at least not for the things I care about—sustainable health systems, cultural preservation, epistemic justice, genuine partnership between state and society. The evidence is there if we're willing to see it.

References

Albert, S. & Porter, J. (2015). "Is 'mainstreaming AYUSH' the right policy for Meghalaya, northeast India?" *BMC Complementary and Alternative Medicine*, 15(1), 288.

Blomkamp, E. (2021). "Systemic design practice for participatory policymaking". *Policy Design and Practice*, 4(1), 12-31. https://doi.org/10.1080/25741292.2021.1887576

Deaton, A. & Cartwright, N. (2018). "Understanding and misunderstanding randomized controlled trials". *Social Science & Medicine*, 210, 2-21.

Kudlu, C. (2025). "From desired futures to market realities: examining policy imaginaries and strategies in the globalization of Ayurveda". *Frontiers in Human Dynamics*, 7, 1549341. https://doi.org/10.3389/fhumd.2025.1549341

Lambert, H. (2015). "The cultural logic of Indian medicine: Prognosis and etiology in Rajasthani popular therapeutics". In *Medical Pluralism in Contemporary India* (pp. 85-110). Routledge.

Mintrom, M. & Einfield, C. (2024). "Co-design in policymaking: From an emerging to an embedded practice". *Policy Sciences*, 57(1), 45-67. https://doi.org/10.1007/s11077-024-09550-9

Mishra, A. (2018). "Persistence of traditional health practices: A study of rural India". *International Journal for Equity in Health*, 17(1), 177. https://doi.org/10.1186/s12939-018-0889-4

Nandi, S. & Schneider, H. (2014). "Addressing the social determinants of health: A case study from the Mitanin (community health worker) programme in India". *Health Policy and Planning*, 29(suppl. 2), ii71-ii81.

Patwardhan, K., Katoch, D., & Nagarkar, A. (2023). "India and its pluralistic health system: A new philosophy for Universal Health Coverage". *The Lancet Regional Health - Southeast Asia*, 9, 100153. https://doi.org/10.1016/j.lansea.2022.100153

Pritchett, L. & Sandefur, J. (2015). "Learning from experiments when context matters". *American Economic Review: Papers & Proceedings*, 105(5), 471-475. https://doi.org/10.1257/aer.p20151016

Scott, J. C. (1998). *Seeing like a state: How certain schemes to improve the human condition have failed.* Yale University Press.

Scott, K., Shanker, S., & Singh, R. (2019). "Community health workers' performance and accountability: A qualitative study exploring the role of community health workers within the health system in India". *Human Resources for Health*, 17(1), 1-15. https://doi.org/10.1186/s12960-019-0358-7

Sharma, N. K., Kumar, R., Angmo, D., Dolma, P., Chaudhary, S., & Kumar, V. (2025). "Traditional therapeutic practices in the Himalayan heartland of Kinnaur, Himachal Pradesh, India: A qualitative exploration". *Journal of Ethnobiology and Ethnomedicine*, 21(1), 5. https://doi.org/10.1186/s13002-025-00742-9

Perspective 12

Polarity: The Sufi Way to Health

Rhea D'Souza

Kabila Consulting, Mumbai

Background

Contemporary health systems, human bodies, and inner lives are frequently approached through linear, solution-oriented models that seek to eliminate tension and arrive at stable outcomes. Yet, both contemporary systems theory and ancient wisdom traditions suggest that many enduring challenges are not problems to be solved but polarities to be managed over time. This article proposes an integrative framework for healing grounded in Barry Johnson's polarity management theory and enriched by Sufi metaphysics, Indian philosophical symbolism, and contemporary understandings of complex systems. By reframing health challenges as dynamic relationships between interdependent forces, this approach offers a more sustainable and humane model of healing—one that emphasises rhythm, balance, and conscious movement rather than control and resolution. From this perspective, polarity is not a limitation of health systems or human experience. It is the very condition that makes sustainable healing possible.

When Health Is Treated as a Problem

Modern medicine has been shaped by industrial logic: identify the malfunction, isolate the cause, apply the intervention, eliminate the symptom. When such approaches succeed, they can be lifesaving. When they fail, frustration often follows—directed toward the body, the healthcare system, or the individual. What if the frustration arises not from inadequate intervention but from misframing? Many persistent health challenges are treated as problems to be solved when they are, more accurately, polarities to be managed over time. My entry into this understanding emerged not through theory but through lived experience. I repeatedly attempted to resolve what I perceived as contradiction—analysis versus intuition, structure versus flow. Each attempt to "choose one side" intensified internal strain, manifesting as physical tightness and emotional holding. Relief came not from resolution but from reframing. When I recognised this tension as a polarity rather than a problem, something softened. Both sides could coexist. The pressure dissolved. This insight led me to polarity thinking and, more deeply, to the Sufi understanding of life as rhythmic movement between complementary forces.

Human bodies, healthcare organisations, and inner lives are complex adaptive systems. Attempts to privilege one pole—control over trust, activity over rest, intervention over self-regulation—often destabilise the whole. Healing, therefore, may not lie in eliminating tension but in restoring rhythm.

Polarity Management Theory: Barry Johnson's Model

The contemporary conceptual foundation for polarity thinking comes from Barry Johnson, who first articulated the distinction between problems and polarities and developed the Polarity Map® as a practical tool for managing enduring tensions rather than solving them as if they were discrete problems. The Polarity Management framework holds that many complex issues are best understood not as solvable problems but as interdependent pairs of values or goals, each of which has a positive contribution when engaged and a negative cost when overemphasised. As Johnson explains, polarities (also called paradoxes or interdependent pairs) are "sets of opposites that need each other over time" and are ubiquitous in human systems from individual behaviour to teams and organisations. His polarity mapping methodology makes the upsides and downsides of both poles visible, allowing practitioners to maximise benefits while minimising risks. Barry Johnson's Polarity Map provides a structured way to visualise and manage interdependent tensions between two poles, such as activity versus rest. The process involves drawing a simple quadrant grid and filling it collaboratively to reveal upsides, downsides, and action steps.

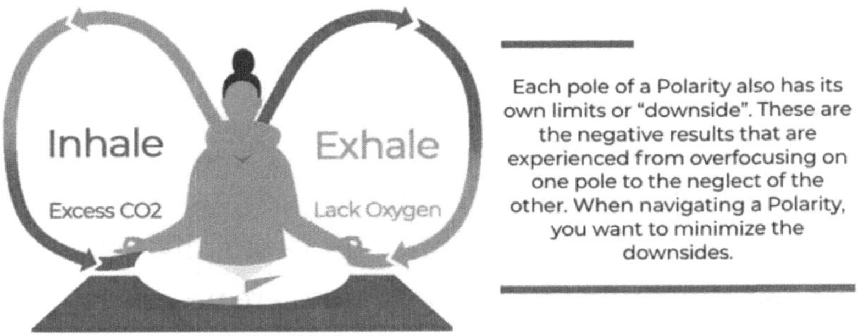

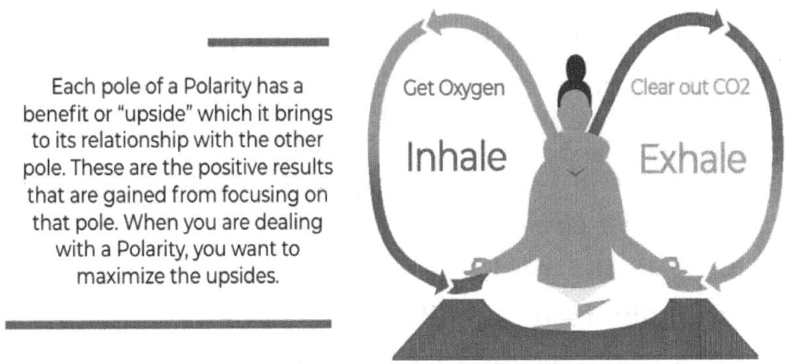

Polarity Map Structure

The map divides into a quadrant grid with two poles (e.g., Pole A on top-left, Pole B on top- right). The upper quadrants list the upsides of each pole (e.g., activity brings a sharp mind and toned body), while the lower quadrants show the downsides of over-focusing on one (e.g., activity overuse leads to burnout; rest overuse leads to dullness). A higher purpose box sits above (e.g., "greater performance") and a deeper fear box below (e.g., "stagnation or exhaustion"). Arrows form an infinity loop, showing natural oscillation between the poles, with diagonals as true opposites (upside of one counters downside of the other).

Step 1: Identify the Issue

Select a persistent challenge that has no single "right" solution but involves ongoing trade-offs, like stability versus innovation. Ensure both sides are necessary over time and that you can influence them.

Step 2: Name the Poles

Draw a 2x2 grid (plus sign dividing it). Label the top-left and top-right quadrants with neutral, positive pole names (e.g., "Stability" and "Change"). These represent the two opposing yet interdependent values.

Step 3: List Upsides and Downsides

Brainstorm positives of the first pole (e.g., predictability from stability) in the upper-left quadrant; positives of the second (e.g., growth from change) in the upper-right; negatives of over-focusing on the first (e.g., stagnation) in the lower-left; and negatives of over-focusing on the second (e.g., chaos) in the lower-right.

Step 4: Add Purpose and Fear

Above the grid, write a "Higher Purpose" that both poles serve (e.g., sustained success). Below, note the "Deeper Fear" of imbalance (e.g., failure or burnout).

Draw curved arrows in an infinity loop connecting the quadrants to show natural tension flow.

Step 5: Develop Actions and Warnings

For each upper quadrant, list 1-3 actionable steps to maximise upsides (e.g., "Schedule quarterly reviews"). Under each lower quadrant, add early warning signs of downside risks (e.g., "Rising staff turnover"). Monitor and act to stay on in the upsides.

Key Guidelines

Pole names should avoid negative connotations (e.g., use "Stability" instead of "Rigid"). Convert "from-to" statements into two poles, such as "from chaos to stagnation" becoming "Change" and "Stability". Keep them concise, ideally one or two words, to fit the map's top quadrants.

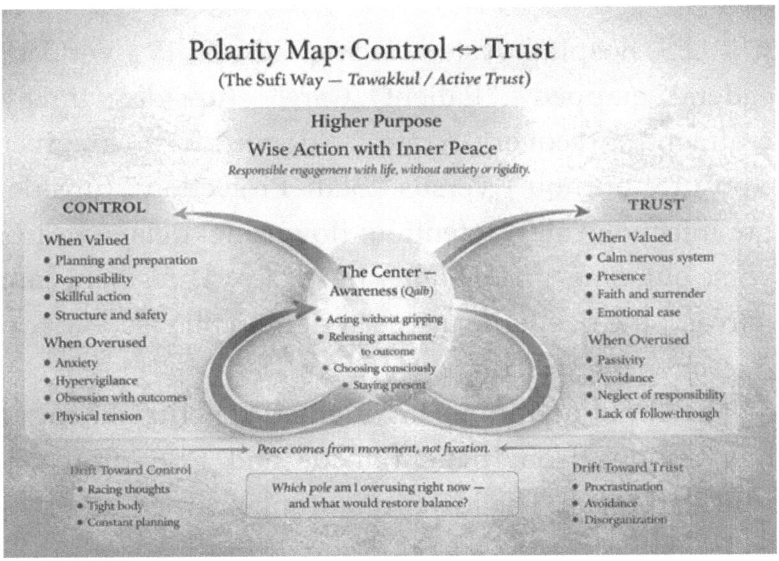

Health Examples

Activity vs. Rest
Nutrition vs. Indulgence
Prevention vs. Treatment

Case Study

Barry Johnson's Polarity Management offers a practical example in addressing actual health issues like patient safety versus staff safety in hospital emergency departments. This tension arises during high-pressure scenarios, such as pandemics or surges, where prioritising one pole risks the other. This polarity exists in many other places where Patient and Caregiver are seen as two opposite receivers.

Case Context

In a U.S. hospital system facing COVID-19 overload, leaders mapped "Patient Care" (upside: timely treatment, recovery rates; downside: caregiver exposure, burnout) versus "Staff Protection" (upside: low infection rates, retention; downside: delayed care, worse outcomes). The higher purpose was resilient care delivery; the deeper fear was systemic collapse.

Map Application

The upper quadrants highlighted benefits like rapid interventions from patient focus and PPE protocols from staff focus. The lower quadrants warned of errors from exhaustion or queues from over-caution. Actions included rotating shifts for balance and real-time dashboards for monitoring; infinity arrows showed ongoing flow.

Outcomes

The staff applied the map in daily huddles, reducing burnout by 25 per cent while maintaining care standards, proving polarity thinking fosters "both/and" solutions for real health crises over "either/or" failures.

Polarity in Healthcare Systems

Healthcare organisations exemplify polarity-rich environments. Integrated health systems must simultaneously manage competing yet necessary demands: cost and quality, physician autonomy and administrative coordination, standardisation and individualised care. Attempts to privilege one side invariably destabilise the system, leading to burnout, inefficiency, or erosion of trust. As documented in healthcare management literature, polarity management enables organisations to value both poles while mitigating the downsides of overuse, supporting adaptability in complex and evolving contexts.

Polarity vs. the Single-Solution Trap in Health

A problem has a solution. A polarity has no final answer—only wise, ongoing management.

When health is polarised, we :

- Choose one side (a diet, a treatment, a philosophy)
- Reject its opposite
- Expect permanence
- Become disappointed when the body inevitably changes again

The Sufi way does not ask, "Which side is right?" It asks, "What rhythm is missing?" This is where polarity maps become essential, not to fix health but to inquire into it.

Why Polarity Maps are Needed in Healing

A polarity map helps us to:

- Name the two essential forces at play
- Honour the gifts of both
- Recognise the cost of over-identifying with either

Used this way, polarity maps shift the health inquiry from: "How do I eliminate this?" to "What balance is asking to be restored?"

Polarised vs. Polarity Thinking (Key Distinction)

Polarisation hardens the heart. In contrast, polarity keeps it turning. Polarised thinking is either/or, where one side is right, tension must be eliminated, and final solutions are sought, creating rigidity. It views health as a battle, driven by blame and fear, control and certainty. Polarity thinking is both/and, where both sides are necessary, tension must be managed, and ongoing movement is accepted, encouraging flow. It views health as a relationship, driven by curiosity and learning, balance and responsiveness.

Health "Problems" that are Actually Polarities

Many common health challenges are misframed as problems, when they are more accurately understood as polarities asking for balance.

Fatigue - Activity ↔ Rest

Fatigue is often treated as weakness or failure, something to override or suppress. From a polarity perspective, fatigue signals an imbalance between exertion and restoration.

- Activity brings purpose and engagement.
- Rest brings repair and integration.

Excessive activity leads to burnout, while excessive rest leads to stagnation.

Insight: Fatigue is not the enemy; it is a teacher calling the soul back into rhythm.

Chronic Pain - Holding ↔ Letting Go

Pain is often approached as something to be eliminated at all costs. Yet, chronic pain frequently reflects excessive holding—physical, emotional, or spiritual—without adequate release.

- Holding offers structure and protection.
- Letting go allows flow and adaptability.

Too much holding creates rigidity, while too much letting go creates collapse.

Insight: Pain becomes the body's *dhikr*—repeating the message that softness is missing.

Anxiety - Control ↔ Trust

Anxiety is commonly framed as a nervous system malfunction. Polarity thinking reveals it as over-identification with control and future management.

- Control provides responsibility and planning.
- Trust offers surrender and presence.

Too much control breeds fear, while too much trust without action leads to passivity.

Insight: Peace arises not by abandoning effort but by releasing attachment to outcome — *tawakkul,* active trust.

The following Sufi saying reiterates this: "Tie your camel, and then trust in God."

Immune & Autoimmune Conditions - Defence ↔ Tolerance

The immune system is often described as either "too weak" or "too strong". Health, however, depends on discerning self from other without aggression.

- Defence protects survival. · Tolerance maintains harmony.

Over-defence turns inward (autoimmunity), while over-tolerance leads to vulnerability.

Insight: Healing here mirrors spiritual maturity—strength without hostility, boundaries without rejection.

Ibn Arabi's quote reiterates this: "Every constriction is a call to expansion."

This approach aligns deeply with the Sufi understanding of healing as return, not conquest.

The Sufi Tradition: Polarity as Lived Wisdom

Long before polarity was formalised as a systems model, the Sufi tradition articulated a lived understanding of balance as central to human flourishing. Sufism does not seek to resolve opposites but to circulate between them with awareness.

Central to Sufi metaphysics is the dynamic interplay of divine qualities, often expressed as:

- *Jamāl* (Beauty, mercy, softness)
- *Jalāl* (Majesty, strength, rigour)

Neither quality is sufficient alone. Excess Jamāl leads to passivity and dissolution, while excess Jalāl leads to hardness and fragmentation. Spiritual maturity—and by extension, health—arises through the rhythmic integration of both.

Sufi practice emphasises tawakkul (active trust): disciplined effort coupled with surrender of outcome. This precisely mirrors the polarity of control and trust, a recurring theme in both anxiety and healing.

Jesus (ʿĪsā), in the Sufi tradition, is regarded as a teacher of inward balance and integration. His teachings consistently point toward a way of living that holds apparent opposites in relationship rather than resolving them through rigid adherence to one side.

Statements such as "Whoever wants to save their life will lose it, and whoever loses their life will find it" (Matthew 16:25) articulate a polarity between holding on and letting go, effort and surrender. Similarly, "Be wise as serpents and innocent as doves" (Matthew 10:16) presents wisdom and innocence not as alternatives but as complementary qualities.

From a Sufi perspective, these teachings align with the understanding that truth does not reside at extremes but emerges through conscious movement between them. In this sense, Jesus' teachings reinforce the polarity-based view of health and human flourishing as dynamic, relational, and sustained through balance rather than resolution.

Importantly, Sufism can be understood as a form of longitudinal phenomenological research, developed through centuries of embodied practice, observation, and transmission. Its relevance to healing lies in its insistence that inner division manifests as outer disorder, including physical symptoms.

The Centre: The Sufi Key to Healing

In polarity maps, the centre is where awareness lives. In Sufism, the centre is the heart that turns.

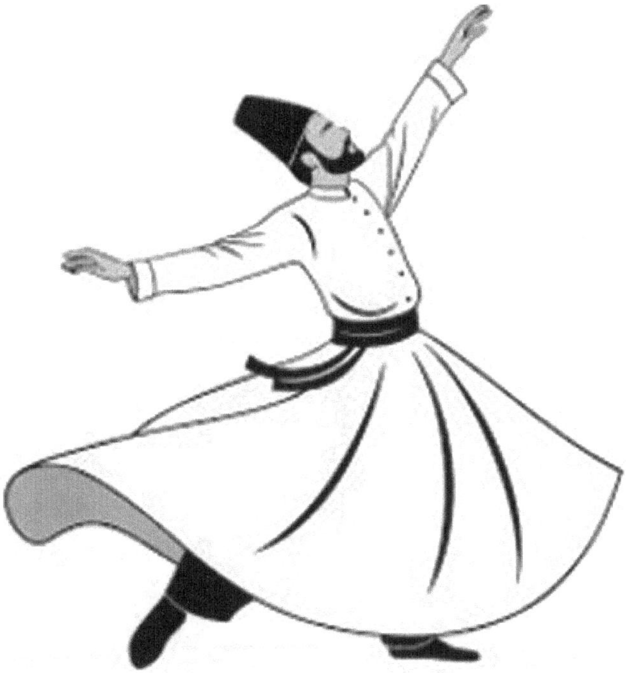

The centre is not still because nothing moves.
The centre is still because everything moves through it.

From this centre, health is not controlled—symptoms are not enemies, the body is listened to, not dominated. Healing becomes an ongoing conversation, not a final answer.

Indian Philosophical Foundations: Shiva and Rhythmic Balance

The logic of polarity is also deeply embedded in Indian philosophical traditions. The figure of Shiva, particularly as Nataraja, the cosmic dancer, embodies the universe as rhythmic movement rather than static form. Shiva's damaru (hourglass drum) symbolises creation and dissolution, expansion and contraction, sound and silence.

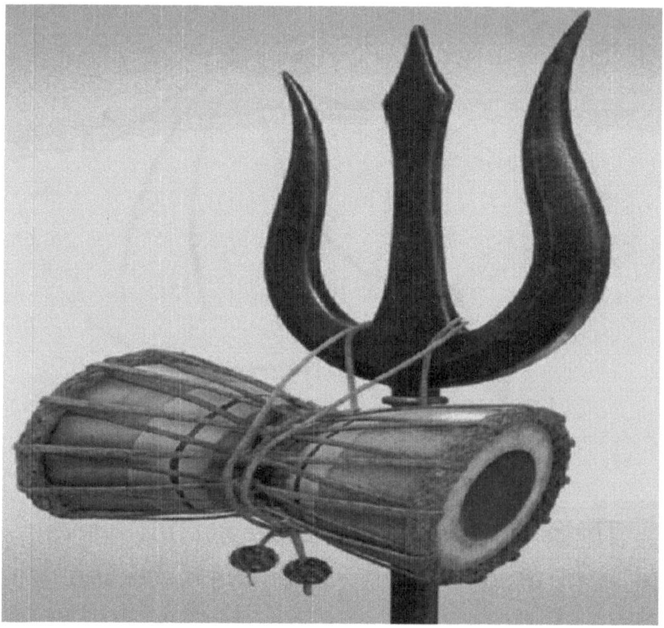

The shape of the damaru—narrow at the centre and expanding toward both ends—visually echoes the structure of a polarity map. Reality is sustained not by equilibrium but by oscillation around a living centre.

Resonance with Contemporary Science

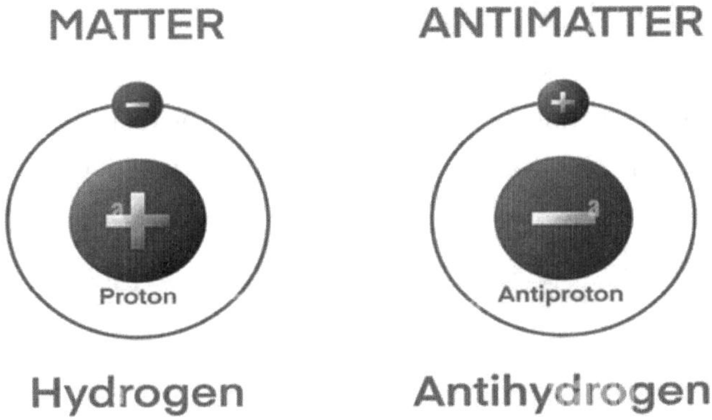

Modern complexity science and physics further support this understanding. In quantum theory, phenomena such as matter and antimatter or wave–particle duality reveal reality as constituted by interdependent opposites arising from the same underlying field. Stability emerges not from dominance of one force but from regulated tension between complementary dynamics.

Living systems—biological, psychological, and social—function similarly. Attempts to optimise a single variable often destabilise the whole. Health, therefore, is not a fixed state but a process of ongoing regulation.

Implications for Healing Practice

When applied to healing, polarity thinking reframes many so-called health problems as signals of imbalance rather than failures to be eradicated. Fatigue reflects imbalance between activity and rest; anxiety reflects imbalance between control and trust; chronic pain reflects imbalance between holding and letting go.

From this perspective, healing is not achieved by eliminating tension but by learning to hold it gracefully. The role of the healer shifts from fixing to facilitating balance, allowing the system—body, mind, or organisation—to self-correct through restored rhythm.

Conclusions

We are living in the aftermath of the industrial era, shaped by mechanised ways of seeing the world, including the human body. In this paradigm, systems are treated as machines—designed to be optimised, controlled, and repaired through linear intervention. While this approach has produced important advances, it has also narrowed our understanding of living systems. The body is not a machine but a living, breathing system, sustained through rhythmic processes of inhalation and exhalation, activation and recovery, engagement and rest. Health, therefore, cannot be reduced to static targets or single interventions. It must be understood as dynamic regulation within a complex system. Polarity thinking offers a framework for this shift, recognising that life is maintained through the continuous movement between complementary forces. The Sufi way, with its emphasis on rhythm, presence, and balance, provides a coherent philosophical and experiential foundation for relating to the body as a living system rather than a mechanism to be controlled.

Across systems theory, spiritual traditions, and contemporary science, a shared insight emerges: life sustains itself through polarity. Attempts to collapse complexity into singular solutions may offer short-term relief but undermine long-term coherence.

Polarity management provides a practical framework for navigating this reality. The Sufi tradition offers the ethical and experiential grounding to hold it with humility and compassion. Indian cosmology and modern physics alike affirm that balance is not stasis, but movement. Health, therefore, is not found at one pole. It is found in the dance between them.

Tu ka Tu – Sufi poetry by Kabir
(English Translation)

In every body, there is my lord,
No vessel is empty - I revere that body which reveals the lord.
O God, your divinity
Pervades everybody,
Like the unseen red
In the green henna leaf.
Do you see the difference, O wise one! Always engage in good deeds,
Be it flowers or branches, in this whole world wherever I look, I see you.

As an elephant, you become huge,
And in an ant, you are tiny,
As a mahout, you sit on top,
And the driver is you, only you.
With thieves you become a thief,
You are in scoundrels too,
You are the one who robs and runs,
The cop who nabs is also you, only you.
With givers you become a giver-You are among the paupers too!
As a beggar you go begging-The donor too is you, only you!
In man and woman only "the one" resides,
Who in this world could call them two.
As a child, you start to cry,
The care-taker is also you, only you.
In water, earth and life you are present - Wherever I look, I see you, only you!
Says Kabir, listen seeker - I have found a guru,
as is, where is.

The enduring relevance of Kabir lies in his articulation of a relational ontology that predates contemporary polarity theory yet mirrors it with remarkable clarity. In verses such as Tu ka tu, Kabir does not advocate the negation of one pole in favour of another; rather, he gestures toward a mode of knowing in which apparent opposites—self and other, effort and surrender, knower and known—are held in dynamic relation until their separation loses coherence. This "both/and" orientation, central to Sufi metaphysics, is not presented as an abstract doctrine but as an embodied realisation. That Kabir's words continue to resonate centuries later suggests that polarity is not merely a cultural construct but a structural artefact, one that we need to wake up to and embody, to remain healthy.

References

Johnson, B. (1996). *Polarity Management: Identifying and Managing Unsolvable Problems*. Amherst, MA: HRD Press.

Suter, E., Oelke, N. D., Adair, C. E., & Armitage, G. D. (2009). "Ten key principles for successful health systems integration". *Healthcare Quarterly*, 13, 16–23.

Uma Shankari, B. & Franklin, A. S. (2012). "Polarity management in healthcare systems: Challenges and opportunities". *Journal of Contemporary Research in Management*, 7(1), 49–55.

Ernst, C. W. (2011). *Sufism: An Introduction to the Mystical Tradition of Islam*. Boston: Shambhala.

The Holy Bible. Gospel of Matthew 10:16; 16:25.

Chittick, W. C. (1989). *The Sufi Path of Knowledge: Ibn al-Arabi's Metaphysics of Imagination*. Albany: SUNY Press.

"Shiva. Iconography of Nataraja and the Damaru". https://www.hinduamerican.org/blog/nataraja-cosmic-dancer-symbolism

Zimmer, H. (1946). *Myths and Symbols in Indian Art and Civilization*. Princeton: Princeton University Press.

Coomaraswamy, A. K. (1957). *The Dance of Shiva*. New York: Noonday Press.

Capra, F. (1996). *The Web of Life: A New Scientific Understanding of Living Systems*. New York: Anchor Books.

Prigogine, I. & Stengers, I. (1984). *Order Out of Chaos*. New York: Bantam Books.

Bohm, D. (1980). *Wholeness and the Implicate Order*. London: Routledge.

Illich, I. (1976). *Limits to Medicine: Medical Nemesis*. London: Marion Boyars.

Perspective 13

How Do We Design a Health System that Allows for Integration of Plural Knowledge?

Prof (Retd) Ritu Priya Mehrotra
Jawaharlal Nehru University

The Challenge

When we look at designing health systems with pluralism, bringing in multiple systems of knowledge, we face a big challenge. The field of health systems research and design is, globally, premised primarily on modern biomedical knowledge as the sole basis for building health systems (Priya, 2022a). In India, integrating the formal, modern, and traditional systems of knowledge is a challenge we have been discussing and trying to address for over 100 years but in a way oriented to the global discourse. Further, the present government health policy discussion focuses only on formal institutional structures, whether of modern or traditional knowledge systems, whereas the real-world health system has both formal and informal dimensions (2023b). The informal has hardly been acknowledged in policy circles, except to denigrate and ridicule it. Civil society and academia have documented and analysed all three systems of knowledge and even attempted integration, but their efforts have not been able to influence policies adequately in this direction (Priya, 2023a).

During the time when the British were ruling India, the debate on integration was already on, and it has continued right up to today. Just before COVID and during COVID, the NITI Aayog attempted to bring together several health system designers for workshops to figure out how to create an integrated health system. I understand that this exercise could not come up with a way to do it. Moreover, that is a puzzle. In today's day and age, with sustainability science, transdisciplinary research, and other such frontiers of science that have opened up from the classical positivist science to much more collaborative science, one would expect that experts in the country would have come up with some feasible ideas. In our kind of context, where we have eight officially recognised health systems, while we should have, by now, worked out their respective places in the system, we obviously have not. I will spell out what the challenges are as I understand them, having engaged with the Ministry of AYUSH and with what we teach in academic public health and health systems, and thereby identify the gaps because of which we are not able to think of integrative systems.

A Comprehensive Integrative Health System

Health systems are complex because of the many factors shaping health and the many elements that constitute health care. All of these components will need to integrate the various forms of knowledge (Priya, 2021; 2023c).

Integrative Self-Care

It is clear that we need integrative self-care. If we just think about what our families do when we suffer from an illness, we realise that, in fact, most of us adopt integrative self-care. However, there are challenges present as well. I think we are all aware of the changes happening in our lifestyles, the environmental pollution around us, changes in disease patterns, and so on. We now have more diverse sources of information, from our families and community to the internet. Therefore, we do need some deep thinking around the changes required in self-care.

Integrative Patient Care at Primary, Secondary, and Tertiary Levels

However, beyond integrative self-care, we need integrative patient care. Today, most of the big corporate private hospitals have units of Ayurveda and Homeopathy, and are now attempting to work together. Therefore, this realisation at the patient care level is already there and is coming into institutional practice. While it has been there in various ways all the time, it is now getting institutionalised in some form. But how does it happen at the primary, secondary, and tertiary levels? Everybody considers integrative care to be good, thinking that communities can do what they want at the primary level. But if there is anything a little more serious, then it must go to the dominant form. However, if it's reaching tertiary hospitals now, it shows that there is a growing realisation of the need at each of these levels, which the practitioners and managers of the dominant knowledge form also recognise.

Integrative Public Health

We need an integrative public health system because the preventive system that everybody spoke about earlier gets institutionalised through public health practice in the dominant modern system. But it doesn't seem to have enough thought to pick up all the other knowledge systems that are there.

We must ask the question, "And what would integrative public health do?" It would have to move well beyond health service systems and into looking at questions such as: What kind of food do we need? What kind of food processing do we need? What kind of dietary guidelines are given all the time? We are all taught in school what a balanced diet is. Should dietary guidelines be somewhat different and more flexible by considering diverse knowledge systems? What kind of living and working conditions are most conducive to health? What is it that we need to introduce in school education and higher education, including medical education, if we want integrative systems? Sports, exercise, leisure time—how do we want to design these for our children, adults, and the elderly? All these are issues for public health and for health at large.

Hence, we'll have to look at a whole spectrum of things if we want to look at it as integrative public health, where, again, we don't think of only the modern dominant models that are before us but also of all the wisdom and knowledge that we have had with us as a society for a long, long time. Fortunately, in our society, we still have some people with prior knowledge and engaged in the practice of these as living traditions.

So, what should we consider when designing integrated health systems? If we want to design and think of a health system as a comprehensive health system, we'd have to work on all three dimensions: integrative self-care, integrative patient care, and integrative public health (Priya, 2023c).

Relatively Recent Issues

Environmental Degradation

Environmental pollution is the big, relatively new, entrant on the public health scene, with a new meaning in the last 100 to 200 years. How do we mitigate that? What are the measures we would need to do that? Traditional knowledge may not provide all the answers, as some contaminants are new, and their quantities in the environment are recent problems. However, the traditional local materials and low-consumption lifestyles certainly provide pointers to how we can deal with the problem at its root. Context-specific rules of waste disposal and sanitation are also available in traditional systems as cultural norms. However, a challenge for traditional systems is the likely effect of the pollutants on the herbal medicines they use, one that has not been adequately recognised or addressed (Priya, 2022b).

Community Action and Social Cohesion for Health

Collectivisation of communities, which used to exist almost naturally, has now become an issue for health systems. Our social fabric is not as robust as it used to be, and there is clearly a decrease in social cohesion within families and between families, between communities, and in society at large. Therefore, this needs to be brought back again for community well-being and certainly for community health action.

Vantage Point for Designing Health Systems

One challenge when we talk about designing health systems is the need for a planned design process. When dealing with top-down institutional structures, how can we incorporate the contextual and diverse bottom-up experiences and needs? It's not one universal model that we can create, and, therefore, we require decentralised processes that can achieve this.

So, how do we establish that link between bottom-up planning and what that requires, and the top-down institutional structure, which is going to plan and create the designs for society? How do we manage this challenge at the societal level today, as the state becomes the major planner and designer of our societies? What have been the challenges to this (Priya, 2025)?

A major issue is that modern science's positivist nature claims there is only one truth, which only science can provide. In other words, only the modern scientific method provides that one truth, which is universally valid and applicable. And this is something that is drilled into us by our educational system from school onwards.

At the time of independence, our planners had to negotiate the difficulties associated with that technological paradigm. At that time, as a society, we were in awe of the technological paradigm—there was medical science and technology, newly developed antibiotics, painkillers, etc., all of which were magic bullets. Therefore, there was much awe of modern systems, which the planners saw as the basic knowledge system we needed to adopt and spread. The committees which developed our health systems, such as the Bhore Committee, almost exclusively comprised modern medical doctors. It decreed that other systems must just die out; we don't need them now that we have the modern scientific system. However, fortunately, because our political and cultural context required it, all the other systems survived even institutionally (Priya, 2023d). Even the committees which were meant to study other knowledge systems and how to integrate them, such as the Chopra Committee, all thought that integration eventually had to be done with modern medicine as the reference point, and everything would integrate within it. In other words, we will see what is good in others and integrate it, the idea being there can be only one science, and even if we integrate various knowledge systems, we have to create that one integrated science.

A major question is how we want to see integration. Even today, when, for example, the National Rural Health Mission does co-location of various systems, i.e., in one PHC or one hospital, we have people of Ayurveda, Unani, Siddha, or Homeopathy and so on, along with the modern system, one would imagine it would mean allowing dialogue and experience-sharing cross talk. It would mean integrative patient care. But no dialogue takes place because we are in the mode of integrating everything into modern medicine. So, these doctors, at best, if they have their own system's medicines in the PHC and hospital, may use them, but even then they are required to practise the allopathy that is part of the modern system as National Health Programmes for disease control.

Is that the integration we want at the patient care

level? Or is it that we would want each knowledge tradition to grow with its own principles and practise in its own wisdom, with its own genius? We then have eight different systems being practised simultaneously and being allowed to do their own research, to grow, to develop their own educational systems, etc., which is what we have officially adopted in practice, as distinct from China, which has done a much more amalgamative exercise. We still have this diversity of eight systems, their councils, their separate medical colleges, and so on. Therefore, I think that is one positive which we already have in our system.

Now, one way would be to go the way the dominant planning process goes. We start top-down. We say we have so many Ayurveda colleges and so many Homeopathy colleges, but we need so many more because the population needs so many doctors. Therefore, let's build so many more hospitals, medical colleges, and so on, and then we try to see how we fill this shortfall.

The other way is to say what it is that people do, which knowledge system they use, why they use it, and thereby see what we need from there upwards and what challenges people face. For example, you'll find when we talk of home remedies now, people say they don't have the plants that they used to have around them—the forests have gone far away, and, therefore, they can't find those plants. Some community healers continue to be there, while some have migrated out of the villages or their children have stopped practising because it wasn't legitimate to practice. Therefore, how we now handle these situations would become part of what we need to plan for and design for. Therefore, how we coordinate between these situations and prioritise would be issues that we need to look at.

The Epistemological and Ontological Differences

The positivist modern science and its claim of universality and singularity of knowledge is one major stream of thought that we have to break out of. In the present times, sustainability science is helping us do that. The earlier traditions of health and medical knowledge, too, accept the idea of diverse knowledge systems co-existing, which were in dialogue with each other in earlier times and drew from the strengths of the other.

Another basis of modern bio-medicine is the Descartian body-mind divide, putting in separate silos the physical body as biological and the mind as psychological. By this logic, the environment was considered to some extent, but the social and spiritual dimensions had to be sifted out completely in order to know the biological body. There are now elements in the frontiers of modern science and modern medicine today which are attempting to correct this kind of divide between body and mind. For instance, the bio-psycho-social approach is being propagated in clinical practice to address all health problems. Systems biology is also breaking the silos. In conventional bio-medicine, only some diseases, like asthma and allergies, were labelled as psychosomatic, but the rest were all categorised as either biological or pyschological—body is body, and mind is mind. Now we know that's not true. There's so much that makes them closely interknitted. Homeopathy, of course, has always taken that into account, as do the basic precepts of yoga and other knowledge traditions.

The common practice of modern bio-medicine is currently called "conventional medicine" in public health and health systems research. While writing a popular article in Hindi, I realised when you say conventional medicine, it becomes *paramparic chikitsa*—that's the only term we have for it. Hence, traditional and conventional are both *paramparic* because conventional bio-medicine now has been practised across the world for at least 100 years. A 100-year history makes it something which is conventional or traditional. It is not ancient tradition, but it is something which is widely accepted and practised as a stream of knowledge. Therefore, this is one whole area of the knowledge systems and how we view them—as "modern" and "traditional" or as various traditions of knowledge that co-exist. The traditional knowledges were born in earlier time periods, while the modern is the most recent. All are changing and adapting to modern/contemporary times.

The second major challenge arises from the political economy of health care. The medical-industrial complex, currently the largest economic sector after IT and possibly defence, along with its associated patent regime, treats innovation and research as individual phenomena, granting ownership of specific knowledge to either individuals or industries. We are then trying to fit traditional knowledge into that regime. In what has been a fascinating process, the World Intellectual Property Rights Organization (WIPO) has just signed an international treaty (WIPO, 2025). The treaty was debated for over 20 years, with intense discussions occurring between two opposing sides. They were called Group A and Group B. Group A comprised the high-income countries and their pharma industry. On the other side was China, India, Africa, and Latin American countries as Group B. The two were battling several kinds of issues on what to sign. The most contentious issue which was being debated was: should they mandatorily declare where they got the original knowledge from (Javed et al., 2020)? Till the 1950s, most drugs came from traditional medicine and its knowledge and then were converted into molecules and pharma products claimed as modern medicine. Now there has been a return to bioprospecting to find these because it's easy. The knowledge of the community is already there. All that has to be done is to work in the lab to find the effective molecule and make it into a pharmaceutical product. Other processes to identify/produce new drugs are more cumbersome and time consuming—picking up random chemicals and trying to work out what their medical effect could be, or attempting to develop new molecules/particles for specific medical purposes.

The debate on the WIPO treaty text mentioned

earlier had two issues I wish to highlight here: one, it included mandatory disclosure of source of knowledge, and two, it actually had a clause which said that those who use this knowledge—for example, the pharma industry—will have to do some innovation with it to get a patent, which would likely be to pick up the active molecule from the plant used traditionally and make that into a drug. In doing that, the clause was that those who use that knowledge must be cognizant of work in consonance with the culture from which it came. Now that would have meant a completely different thing if every box of a medicine had to say: "This came from the tribes of Kerala, such and such", "This came from Odisha, this came from Australia", and so on. It would start questioning modern science's supremacy because here this is what has created that supremacy—that they came with magic bullets for us and saved our lives. This means saying that what you are taking and selling across the world is what you've got from us, and that is not something the countries were ready for. So, it was hotly debated, and finally, it has not been included in the treaty which all countries have signed, including India (WIPO, 2025). The cultural dimension didn't even get discussed. It was just quietly dropped because nobody could think of how the modern medical industry and pharma industry will be able to deal with the cultures of these societies, acknowledge them, and use them in their processes. One cannot imagine how they could address this issue without completely overturning the principles of science. Since it would be a completely different way of handling knowledge/science, it has not been allowed to happen.

This dominance is not limited to the corporate medical industry and what it is doing with pharmaceuticals. In addition to pharmaceuticals and patents, this issue also encompasses medical equipment, medical diagnostics, and medical insurance, which have now significantly entered our country. All of this together becomes the medical industrial complex, and unfortunately, AYUSH is falling into the trap of following, emulating each of these. Our modern medical education is being questioned, and its regulatory mechanism, the MCI, had to be completely modified. That is why we now have a new institution, the National Medical Commission. Across the globe, this model of regulation of self-regulation of medical professionals, which was practised in the 19th and 20th centuries, has now been abandoned. The self-regulation does not seem to have worked. It's been seen that there have been unethical practices everywhere, and, therefore, the bringing in of not only doctors into that regulatory system but also lay persons and other socially active persons has been the mandate everywhere. This is only an indicator of what we are missing out on, but AYUSH now has the same kind of educational institutions modelled on medical college lines. The college graduates are the only officially recognised practitioners today. The ones that were from a practitioner lineage, or *guru–shishya parampara,* are designated as quacks, and in states like Kerala, they're even banned from speaking or practising in public. We are now moving into that kind of a frame where they are getting pushed out.

In the same centralised and standardising vein, the official agency is trying to make one single homogeneous pharmacopoeia (the list of medicines and how they work) of Ayurveda for the country. While Kerala, Banaras, and Jamnagar have different medicines that they use, the homogenisation of ayurvedic pharmacopoeia into one is what is coming in the name of standardisation. So, while the system needs standardisation of some kind, the moot question is how does one still preserve the diversity which we discussed to be critical? If it has to do with rules, guidelines, or delivery of services for mass use, one would need to think of being cognizant of trying to retain that diversity. So, while designing health systems, how we keep even standardisation flexible and open is something we need to deeply think about.

Research Evidence of Efficacy

Part of the knowledge issues problem that is always raised is about the evidence as proof of efficacy, and homoeopathy knows it better than any of the others. Now those who are experienced in terms of sitting on both sides of the debate (which I have been fortunate to be part of) see that a lot of the time, there is solid evidence and data about cure by natural processes. For instance, even in the case of some diseases like TB, there is spontaneous cure in 40 per cent of those who actually manifest TB, i.e., without any drugs. In other words, in 40 per cent of the cases, the body will cure itself. This is what happens when any of us contract any illness—some spontaneous healing occurs—and that is what all systems benefit from. If I believe in Allopathy and I take allopathic medicine, I will believe I got cured because of that, and it reinforces my belief. If I believe in Homeopathy, I will take homeopathic medicine, and I will recover, whether by nature's doing or by the homeopathic medicine, and I will believe it was Homeopathy that did the trick, and, therefore, it reinforces the belief. All practitioners know this. I am sure that the clinical practitioners here will corroborate what I am saying. So this is a great benefit that all practitioners of all systems avail of. Therefore, when we want to actually know objectively whether a medicine works or not, we will have to go beyond just practitioner experience or patient experience because of this reinforcing process. There has to be some objective way by which we identify the effectiveness of any particular drug or regimen, some way of measuring it. The randomised clinical trials (RCTs), as a study design, are helpful in measuring the efficacy. At the same time, one cannot base all decisions on the RCT findings. There is much valid critique of using the RCT findings as a gold standard for "evidence-based medicine". RCT findings are the first base on which we can say that this is something we can use with proven effect for this particular problem. However, we will need to see whether it works in the context in which we want to use it, since it has been tested under a certain set of conditions and may not be similarly effective in another context. So examining this would be the next step. At the same time, one does not want to throw away the baby with the bathwater, i.e., say that we don't see any value in RCTs at all or ignore them even when the data is there. We need to see it as a process by which we can try and understand what is working at the physical level or physical- cum- psychological levels in terms of treating a particular condition. Hence, will it actually work in a particular context or not is the next step of research that needs to be carried out.

In other traditions of health knowledge, such as Ayurveda, one needs to be able to say under which conditions - *sthan, kaal, prakriti* (*mizaj* in Unani medicine)- will it work or not work. This is their strength. However, this holistic principle is, unfortunately, being given up in practice, and that, to my mind, is a major challenge today. It is difficult to comprehend how Ayurveda research can happen without accounting for particularity, and how it could be ensured without taking *prakriti* into account. However, the research, both in academic settings and by the industry that manufactures ayurveda products, is not taking *prakriti* into account. I have sat on ethics committees of an eminent public institute of Ayurveda, and with my very limited understanding of Ayurveda, it was clear to me that none of their research takes into account *prakriti,* a fundamental principle of Ayurveda. When I questioned about this, the faculty's answer was that "we are not doing even our clinical treatment based on prakriti, so why bring it into the research and make it more difficult?" Here I'm arguing for being allowed to do research under the principles of their own knowledge system, while that knowledge system itself is trying to emulate modern medicine and give up its epistemological roots!

That said, there are some very interesting examples where RCT has been done in keeping with the Ayurveda principle. A very well-known study was conducted in Coimbatore on rheumatoid arthritis, where, with Dr Ram Manohar as the lead, they treated some American patients with rheumatoid arthritis, who were not getting better there. These patients were on medicines like anti-cancer drugs and so on for it. They got treated and went back. Officials from the National Institutes of Health (NIH, USA) came to India and asked the Coimbatore team, "Can we study what you're doing? The RCTs require a very strict protocol: this much drug, so much dose will be given, all that is set out earlier and you cannot change it during the study. You can do another study later if you think it was wrong, but that study will have to take only that." The Coimbatore Ayurveda team clearly stated, "We won't change our system of treatment for your study. We don't have one molecule, we don't have one drug. We will keep changing, and the same patient we may be giving five different regimens as we go along. As the patient's condition changes, we will accordingly change our medicine." The NIH team agreed and worked out an RCT design that would compare the efficacy of Ayurveda treatment versus Methotrexate, which was the drug that they were giving. Their protocol dictated that once the drug is given and is being followed up to see various indices and tests, it is done for a certain period of time, say 6 months, and then there is a follow-up for 6 months. The Ayurveda team countered this and said, "We want follow-up for at least 9 to 12 months because we have seen in our patients that initially results are slow. It is at 9 months that real change happens." So the study was done, and at 6 months, Methotrexate and Ayurveda treatment was at par, and at 9 months, the Ayurveda treatment had overshot the Methotrexate results. Now this is an excellent example to show that the NIH had to change its very sacred RCT protocols to keep to the principles of Ayurveda rather than do it the other way round. I always feel so elated whenever I think of this kind of a situation where a dominant system such as the NIH is made to change its entire approach. The way they demonstrated an openness to experiment with another knowledge system has been well recognised. The study was then internationally awarded.

Now, an important question arises: why is this kind of a design not being followed subsequently for assessing the efficacy of other regimens? Now you have a kind of example from which you can learn how RCTs can be designed for AYUSH, keeping the various diversities into account. You could make three arms with three different prakritis if you want and see how the drugs could work. It, of course, increases the sample size you then need, as well as the time and resources. But yet, I would think if Ayurveda wants to stick to its principles, this is one of the basic things that it needs to do in its research. So I was very impressed with the approach of Dr Khamar when he stated that we try and figure out within the entire patient care where it is that we fit our system and where we fit ourselves. Because each system has strengths and limitations, and if one has a general idea of where it fits, then people know. The health-seeking behaviour studies that we have found show that people have worked out, through experience, their rule of thumb for where to go for what problem. Therefore, their rules of thumb clearly indicate where they will go for each specific issue. This topic, of course, requires more detailed discussion at a later time. Those working with communities and patients would certainly know.

Therefore, what I'm pointing out is how we create the bridges between the different systems, between the health care systems and the other systems that we need for preventing and treating health problems, building on the strengths of each knowledge system. There are examples of the same that have been attempted, like the National Rural Health Mission (NRHM) attempting to do co-location. If that can be operationalised to actually mean interaction, then it'll be useful. Those sitting together in one institution should be trained to know when to cross-refer for what diseases – is their colleague from another system of medicine better for this particular patient with this particular condition and, therefore, should be sent there? Some people have worked it out between them. There is an informal cross-referral, but it is not formal. We did a study across 18 states under the

National Rural Health Mission (Priya and Shweta, 2010) and found that cross-referral is happening. More than 50 per cent of allopathic doctors in the public system said they were doing it and that they saw value in other systems. Yet, they wouldn't write it down. They would tell it verbally, but they will not write it because it is considered illegitimate. They wonder whether they're actually being disloyal to their system and, therefore, will not write it. We need to break that and say this is legitimate. But in doing so, there needs to be some caution today. For instance, if the medicines from different systems interact, do we need to change dosages? Do we need to give one early and give one with a gap, or not give one at all and give the other? These are all things that need to be researched (Priya, 2022b). While individuals can do it for themselves, or a small number in a group can figure this out, systemically, if we want integrative systems, we need to carry out organised research with a very open mind to figure out new insights. The herbal medicines today are growing in the same soil and with the same water and air that we know is contaminated. Do the herbs have that purity or that effect, or can they also have negative effects? We need to test that out. So, this kind of research is required.

Initiatives for Integration

Let's examine a few attempts at integration, highlighting their limited scope. While institutions such as the Indian Institute of Integrative Medicine in Jammu are mandated to do so, I'm afraid that, from what I hear, it's largely RCTs on specific AYUSH drugs that are being tried and nothing beyond that. We have community health officers in the Health and Wellness Centres, now called Arogya Mandirs, where they are either nurses or AYUSH doctors who are being given a bridge course in modern medicine to be able to become Community Health Officers. During a consultation when their bridge course was being created, the discussion was on geriatric care, and the proposal was to train the AYUSH doctors in modern forms of geriatric care. I was completely stunned and asked, "Are you going to teach Ayurvedic practitioners to do modern geriatric care?" They replied in the affirmative and added that is what IGNOU's course is going to do, and that is what was designed. So, there are misleading practices occurring under the guise of integration and bridging. There was a clause in the NRHM, which is now called the Indian Public Health Standards (IPHS), that in the sub-centres and PHC compound, local medicinal herbs will be grown. So, it has a powerful possibility, but it hasn't worked out on the ground.

The Quality Council of India is doing certification of local traditional community healers through a very interesting and rigorous process, which is certainly something to be taken up. At the moment, eight or nine states are doing it, but others have not picked this up yet. There has been a suggestion for creating District Health Resource Centres so that they can understand the local traditional knowledge, ensure that the plants they require are being cultivated there, and also interact with the Biodiversity Act and the forest department to ensure that they remain available to the locals. This is critical because our districts themselves are so large they actually require block-level and *taluka*-level centres. At least, district level centres should document this decentralised knowledge, but these are not taken up really. These centres could also coordinate with the local traditional healers and their voluntary certification process (Priya, 2025).

We come back to the question of how to do this kind of a dialogic process across these systems at the informal knowledge level and the textual knowledge level. Can we create something like a University of Integrative Medicine? That was a proposal we gave to the Planning Commission, which was shot down completely. This could be a place which houses each of the eight systems, each having their own medical college, which does research and teaching in their respective system—an integrative institute, which helps to bring them together on particular problems and to figure out how it would be best to do the integration. We did one very small exercise, and Dr Onkar Mittal of Swasthya Hind was a part of that dialogue on diabetes where we took diabetes Type 2 as our problem and included all eight systems' practitioners as well as folk healers. We talked about the pathology, i.e., its process of development, the symptoms, its diagnosis, prevention, and treatment. It was interesting that the prevention that came out was similar for every system—diet and exercise. So basically, all systems had that understanding, and other aspects were sometimes similar and, of course, also different. This kind of a dialogic process was a very enriching experience. Unfortunately, we couldn't follow up on it, but it was an interesting attempt that we made in JNU (Kurian and Ramanand, 2015).

The proposal for an Integrated Standard Treatment Guidelines would be worth developing. We know that each system has its own treatment guidelines. Can we create an integrated one so that people can try the indigenous things at home, and then at a certain point, go to an expert? Can it include which home remedies people can use for which problem, and also how to do so for the best effects? Which system practitioner should be part of the guidelines for people? It should specify that when people reach such symptoms, it is time to consult a physician. It should also give the strengths and limitations of various systems. All the Integrated Standard Treatment Guidelines would be based on rigorous trans disciplinary research.

These are some of the things which are already institutionalised, while some are at the level of ideas yet, and as proposals that need to be taken up at scale. Small attempts have been made by civil society groups and by some states. But there are certainly possibilities today of moving forward on this agenda. However, the problem lies with the understanding of basic science, and it's making a big comeback. Let me also add that there is sustainability science, which is doing more to open up and saying there are multiple ways of looking at any phenomenon. There are medical bio-psycho-social approaches, and there is a comeback to assert science as the classical science, as we understood it. Health systems research and systems design have to be based on stated values and with a combination of top-down and bottom-up vantage points to develop a comprehensive, integrative health system (Priya et al., 2025). So, I think this is politics of knowledge and a battle for knowledge that we need to be part of to create systems that are more democratic and open to plural knowledges, rather than go back to the singular.

References

- Javed, G., Priya, R., & Deepa, V.K. (2020). "Protection of Traditional Health Knowledge: International Negotiations, National Priorities and Knowledge Commons". *Society and Culture in South Asia,* 6(1), 98–120. DOI: 10.1177/2393861719883069
- Kurian, C. M. & Ramanand, R. (2015). *Report of proceedings of the 'Dialogue on Diabetes: Towards Mutual Understanding Amongst Different Systems and Traditions of Health and Healing'* organised by the Trans-Disciplinary Research Cluster on Pluralist Health Care: Knowledge, Technology, Practices and Policy, Jawaharlal Nehru University, July 30-31, 2015.
- Priya, R. (2025). "Turning the Politics of Knowledge Upside Down; Community-Centred

Public Policy for Sustainable Universal Healthcare Systems". In Reddy, S., Vaidyanathan, G., & Sinha, A. (Eds.) *Healthcare for All: Community Action and Public Systems for an Inclusive India.* Routledge, 86-116.

- Priya, R., Das, S., Kuriakose, L. M., Shukla, M., Sarkar, A., Dumka, N. et al. (2025) "The Dialogic Health Systems Research Framework (DHSRF): A tool for facilitating self-criticality, researcher interactions and knowledge management in Health Systems Research & Policy Studies". *PLOS Glob Public Health,* 5(9): e0004209.
- Priya, R., 2023. "Co-producing and Pluralizing Health Knowledge for Re-visiting Development". In *Dreams of a Healthy India: Democratic Health Care in Post-Covid Times,* (eds.) Priya, R. and Hameed, S. Vintage Penguin Random House, India, 2023: 82-102.
- Priya, R. (2023). "An Expanded Health Systems Perspective on Tribal Health Knowledge and Practices: Contemporary Relevance and Challenges", in Reddy, S., Guite, N., and Subedi, B. (Eds.) *Ethnomedicine and Tribal Healing Practices in India: Challenges and Possibilities of Recognition and Integration (eds.),* Springer, Singapore, 2023: 325-346.
- Priya, R. (2023). ""Integrative Health System" beyond "Integrative Medicine": A health system research perspective for "One Nation, One

Health System"". *J Res Ayurvedic Sci 2023*; 7: 35-41. DOI:10.4103/jras.jras_146_22

- Priya, R. (2023d). "The Evolution of Health Policy Over 75 Years". *IIC Quarterly*, Vol. 49, No. 3 & 4, 14-27.
- Priya, R. (Oct. 2022). "Traditional Medicine in Global Health Systems Approaches: A Review that Calls for Drafting of a PHC 2.0 in Traditional Medicine Review", Vol. 2, No. 2, 3-16.
- Priya, R. (2022). "The Role of Traditional Medicine in Public Health". Editorial in the IJPH; 66: 89-90.
- Priya, R. (2021). "Critical Holism as Public Health Theory: Towards a Unifying Framework for Research, Policy and Planning". Dialogue: *Science, Scientists and Society*, Vol. 4, Special Issue on Public Health.
- Priya, R. and Shweta (2010). "Status and Role of AYUSH Services and Use of Local Health Traditions under the NRHM: A Health Systems Study Across 18 States" (co-author: Shweta Awasthi Saxena), National Health Systems Resource Centre, 2010.
- Priya, R., Singh, R., and Das, S.. "Health Implications of Diverse Visions of Urban Spaces: Bridging the Formal-Informal Divide". In Escalante, A. E., Eakin, H., & Garcia, C. M. (eds.) (2021). *Sustainability Challenges for our Urban Futures*. E-book, Lausanne: Frontiers Media SA. doi: 10.3389/978-2-88966-379-8
- WIPO, 2024. https://www.wipo.int/wipolex/en/treaties/textdetails/19849

Perspective 14

Re-Embedding Health in Place, Practice, and Relational Knowledge

James Oliver
RMIT University
Melbourne, Australia

Background

Contemporary public and institutional understanding about holistic health is a positive evolution of rationalist, enlightenment discourse and often invokes pragmatic concepts of integration, balance, and well-being, but without necessarily situating (or relating with) the epistemological and ecological conditions that make such integration possible. This paper reflects that health must be understood as a relational, ecological, and ethical phenomenon rather than merely a biological or instrumental one. Drawing on Gaelic concepts of emplacement, Indigenous research methodologies, improvisational practice, and hyperlocal land-based work (Oliver 2007, 2009, 2021a, b, c.), I propose a remembering (and, therefore, re-embedding) of health (including well-being) within human ecological relations. Central to this remembering is the distinction between instrumental validity and relational validity (c.f. Tuck and McKenzie, 2015), and the claim that sustainable well-being depends upon the restoration of shared ethical responsibility among people, place, and knowledge systems. It is also a form of cognitive justice (Visvanathan, 1997, 2009).

From Instrumental to Relational Health

Modern health systems have achieved extraordinary technicalcapacity. Yet,theproliferationofchronicdisease, mental health distress, ecological anxiety, and social fragmentation suggests that health cannot be reduced to interventionist efficacy alone. While instrumental approaches to health measurement, standardisation, optimisation, and economics are indispensable, they are part of an ontology of "displacement", too—a displacement of relational ecologies within which well-being is emplaced, experienced, and lived.

This short essay proposes that holistic health requires a remembering and re-embedding of human beings within ecological and ethical relations. Health, in this view, is not an isolated state of bodily functioning but an emergent property of situated belonging and relationships—between personhood and communities, between communities and land, and between knowledge systems and power.

In articulating from this proposition, I draw from the spectrum of my professional and emplaced experience of diverse collaborations of practice and research, across varied social contexts of well-being, cultural and policy practice. This includes within my native Gaelic language and philosophy and land-based cultural revitalisation in Scotland, and also through international Indigenous research and creative collaboration, community arts engagement, and improvisational methodologies. While this work is often within its own cultural geography and situatedness, the collaborations and conceptual implications are globally resonant.

"Is the Grass Blue?" (Epistemology and the Experience of Health)

A traditional, colloquial Gaelic phrase asks (when literally translated), "Is the grass blue?"

Now, in the English language, the question appears incorrect. Grass is green. Yet the Gaelic question and expression here does not concern linguistic truth or the chromatic taxonomy of nature (as if that were indeed the true nature of grass); rather, it concerns semantic depth in relational perception. The grass is perceived to be blue-ish (not necessarily how you perceive to be 'blue' in your language either), where blue and green are sometimes the same quality, and in the daily porosity and multi-generational cultural knowledge of that lived quality of encounter, the language honours the way of seeing and knowing, rather than correcting it through linguistic fixedness and analytic categorisation.

This distinction illuminates a broader ontological and epistemological tension between instrumental and relational validity. Instrumental validity prioritises measurable exactitude and technical classification (for scientific coherence and commodification—not implicitly negative, of course). Relational validity prioritises experiential knowledge that is always emerging within a situatedness and emplacement of cultural encounter (also not implicitly negative).

In health discourse, instrumental validity dominates not only for scalable reasons, such as population levels of health outcome, but also for hierarchies of power and economic rationalisation and profit. Further, in the age of digital health hierarchies of biomarkers, diagnostic categories become reduced to treatment by algorithms. Yet, patients' experiences of alienation, loss of meaning, ecological grief, and cultural dislocation can still escape quantification. The "green" of laboratory certainty may obscure the "blue" of lived experience.

Holistic health must hold both registers simultaneously. It must recognise that well-being is not merely the absence of pathology but the presence of meaningful relation.

Situated Knowledge and the Dis-Embedding of Care

Dominant knowledge systems arise from situated positions shaped by histories of power, privilege, and even exclusion (see Haraway, 1985). Biomedical science, despite its universalising aspirations, is historically located within European epistemological traditions. This does not invalidate its achievements, but it does necessitate reflexivity regarding its scope and limits.

Modern institutional systems, including healthcare, often dis-embed practices from their social contexts. Understanding of healthcare becomes linear and procedural; responsibility becomes individualised, which is not to diminish the wonderful professionals and empathy within healthcare. A metaphor I can share from my Gaelic cultural and social memory illustrates this dynamic and ontology (and belief) of progress, where social forces not only challenge cultural norms but also disrupt cultural competence, cultural health, and the dynamic and ontology of social well-being. As a young person at school, one of the first critical cultural works that I felt resonance with was the insight of a poem by Derick Thomson (1987), "Am bodach-rocais" (The Scarecrow). In this, he describes a stranger in a black outfit (the scarecrow) coming with a new knowledge to rebuke and replace the old. The crux of it was that he entered the social circle, approached the communal fire, removed the coals, and placed them one by one onto each individual's chest. The collective flame extinguished, replaced by the fire and zeal of the new revolutionary spirit of individualism (in this case, it was a missionary disrupting and replacing traditional culture and knowledge and it's ecology of care and reciprocity).

In public health terms, moments and legacies of social trauma—colonisation, displacement, economic precarity—become reframed as individual pathology: depression, anxiety, addiction. Structural determinants of health are privatised into personal responsibility. Re-embedding health requires the restoration of communal fires—practices that reconnect care to culture, place, and collective agency.

Dùthchas: Ontological Ethics and Emotional Well-Being

The Gaelic concept of *dùthchas* lies deep in relationships that the dis-embedding and alienation alluded to in the previous section achieved through place-based and cultural dislocations. It resists straightforward translation. Often rendered as "heritage" or "birthright", it more accurately denotes an embodied ontological relation to place and culture—an entanglement of dwelling, inheritance, memory, and responsibility (c.f. Oliver, 2021a, b, c). Dùthchas implies that identity is not merely psychological but ecological. One belongs to land as land belongs to one's history. This is not ownership in a commodified sense; it is ethical emplacement. The erosion of dùthchas through the individualism of privatisation and commodification of land (and related cultural, linguistic, and social dis-embedding through displacement) produces measurable effects on emotional well-being and futures. Communities disconnected from ancestral land relations often experience significant intergenerational traumas that require thinking differently from dominant norms of wellness or cultural health. Thus, emotional well-being cannot be fully understood without attending to ecological belonging.

Hyperlocal Practice and the Global Archipelago

My story here is not one of exceptionalism through specificity of culture or place, and the conceptualising of the "global archipelago" reframes locality. Islands and land are always in relation, with tides and territories, environments and ecologies. The local is always hyper, in the sense that the local is more than just local; it is hyperlocal. Likewise, hyperlocal health initiatives—rooted in specific communities—are simultaneously embedded in planetary dynamics: climate change, migration, economic restructuring, technological transformation. Hyperlocal practice insists on starting with place—specific land histories, languages, and cultural practices. Yet, it does not retreat into parochialism. Rather, it acknowledges interdependence. In healthcare and well-being terms, this suggests that planetary health and community health are inseparable. Ecological degradation, biodiversity loss, and climate instability are not external environmental issues; they are determinants of human well-being.

Re-Commoning: Ceremony as Care, Ethical Relations as Ecology

Cree Indigenous research scholar Shawn Wilson (2008), in *Research Is Ceremony*, articulates research as relational accountability grounded in five principles: relationship, respect, responsibility, reciprocity, relevance. These principles offer a template for rethinking health systems as ethical ecologies. Research, policy, and practice must not only produce outcomes but also sustain relationships. Rationality, in this framing, is not detached calculation but coherence within a web of relations.

As addressed above, modern processes of privatisation and commodification have intensified alienation from land and community resources. In response, movements toward re-commoning seek to restore shared access and collective stewardship and well-being. Within health systems, analogous processes involve community-based participatory research, arts-in-health initiatives, and cross-sector collaboration. These practices resist purely deficit-based models of illness and instead cultivate positive mental health, through openness, creativity, and relational vitality.

When people in place gather to share knowledge with intentional attentiveness, a form of ceremony arises. Ceremony here is not spectacle but heightened relational awareness. It marks the ethical seriousness of encounter. Such initiatives do not reject biomedical care; they supplement and contextualise it. They recognise that well-being emerges through participation in meaningful shared practices. Health co-design processes, when grounded in reciprocity and respect, become ceremonial in this sense. They are not merely technical workshops; they are enactments of collective responsibility.

Conclusion: Toward a Human Ecology of Health

We inhabit a period of profound relational transformation: ecological instability, cultural dislocation, rapid technological change. These shifts challenge inherited assumptions about health and well-being. Holistic health cannot be reduced simply or only to integrative modalities layered atop biomedical frameworks. It requires a reorientation toward human ecological relations, emplacement, and ethical reciprocity, as well as a renewed relationship with the relevance of commoning in a material sense, not as an abstraction or metaphor for equity or justice with health and well-being. To ask what holistic well-being means is to enter that conversation. It is to acknowledge that we are never merely isolated organisms but participants in shared ecological, ontological, and moral worlds. In that dialogical participation across lived experiences and ways of knowing lies the possibility of health. Health emerges not solely from intervention but from relation. It is sustained not only by treatment but also by being and belonging. It flourishes where people, place, and practice remain in dynamic ethical conversation.

References

Capra, F. (1996). *The Web of Life: A New Scientific Understanding of Living Systems*. Anchor Books.

Haraway, D. (1988). "Situated knowledges: The science question in feminism and the privilege of partial perspective". *Feminist Studies* 14(3), 575–599.

Kirmayer, L. J., Gone, J. P., & Moses, J. (2014). "Rethinking historical trauma". *Transcultural Psychiatry*, 51(3), 299–319.

Oliver, J. & Murray, P. (2007). "The Arts, Well-being and Society". *Journal of Public Mental Health* 6(4), 6-11.

Oliver, J. (2009). "Creativity as Openness: improvising health and care situations". *Health Care Analysis* 17 (4), 318-330.

Oliver, J. (2021a). "Acknowledging relations: dùthchas, seanchas and ethical emplacement". In E. Nicolson and G. Meikle (eds.), *The Commonplace Book of ATLAS*. Portree: ATLAS Arts.

Oliver, J. (2021b). "Islandness: articulating and emplacing relationality". In K., Burnett, R. Burnett, & M. Danson (eds.), *Scotland and Islandness: Explorations in Community, Economy and Culture*, 239-248. Oxford: Peter Lang.

Oliver, J. (2021c), "Our Pluriverse and Gàidhealtachd: emplacing ethical relations". *Scottish Affairs*, Vol. 30 (2). Edinburgh: Edinburgh University Press

Meadows, D. H. (2008). *Thinking in Systems: A Primer*. Chelsea Green Publishing.

Rosaldo, R. (1989). *Culture and Truth: The Remaking of Social Analysis*. Beacon Press.

Thomson, D. S. (1987). "Am bodach-rocais (The Scarecrow)". *Nua-bhàrdachd Gàidhlig: Modern Scottish Gaelic Poems*, (ed.) Donald MacAulay. Canongate.

Tuck, E. & McKenzie, M. (2015). "Relational validity and the 'where' of inquiry: place and land in qualitative research". *Qualitative Inquiry*, 21 (7), 633-638.

Visvanathan, S. (1997). *A Carnival for Science: Essays on Science, Technology and Development*. Oxford University Press

Visvanathan, S. (2009). "The search for cognitive justice". *Seminar*, 597. http://www.india-seminar.com/2009/597/597_shiv_visvanathan.htm

Wilson, S. (2008). *Research Is Ceremony: Indigenous Research Methods*. Fernwood Publishing.

World Health Organization. (2022). *WHO global report on social determinants of health equity*. WHO Press.

Author Profiles

Arvindd Narayanan
<Arvindd.narayanan@gmail.com>

Arvindd Narayanan is an acclaimed violinist and a prominent name in the Delhi Carnatic Music circle who has been performing extensively for over two decades. Arvindd is a graded artist of All India Radio and Doordarshan. Arvindd's major learning in music came from Sangeeta Kalanidhi & Padma Bhushan Vidwan Prof. T. N. Krishnan. True to his guru's teachings, Arvindd has imbibed the Gayaki style and brings it out powerfully in his performances. He has performed extensively across India, both as a soloist and as an accompanist to top-graded artists. He also explores innovative collaborations with other genres while retaining the essence of Carnatic tradition. He has also been contributing to *nritya* (dance) and *natak* (drama). He is part of a musical society, *Rudraksham,* working on making Carnatic music more accessible to youth, and a not-for-profit *Pratyusha Foundation,* which works in the field of health, education, and financial inclusion for masses.

Chandrakant B. Desai
<girijanaik345@gmail.com>

Dr Chandrakant Basavaprabhu Desai, also known as Vaidyaraj Dr C. B. Desai, is a distinguished practitioner of Ayurvedic medicine and a member of the Faculty in Ayurvedic & Yunani System of Medicine (M.F.A.M.). Born in 1945 into a family with a 150-year-old tradition of Ayurveda practice, Dr Desai represents the fourth generation of *vaidyas*. He graduated from Aary-Aangl Vaidyak Mahavidyalay, Satara, in 1970 and began his practice, later earning a Diploma in Acupuncture in 1980. With 50 years of experience, Dr Desai has made significant contributions to Ayurveda, with special interests in earthquake studies, astronomy, and the study of customs and traditions. His Ayurvedic work includes the use of Mudra Therapy, acupuncture, acupressure, and integrative therapies for various diseases, including chronic disorders. He has also conducted special studies on *Karnavedhana*, ear acupuncture, nose piercing, and the use of specific leaves in Agnikarma. Dr Desai's work extends beyond Ayurveda. He is a lifetime member of the Karnataka History Congress and has researched the date of Sharangadhara based on total solar eclipses. He has also compiled a collection of manuscripts, stamps, and coins from around the world. Dr Desai has delivered numerous talks on Ayurveda and related subjects and has received several awards, including the Ayurved Praveena and the Vaidya Bhushana. His work and dedication have made him a respected figure in the field of Ayurveda and beyond.

R. V. Giridhar
<girisidhubvm@gmail.com>

R. V. Giridhar is CEO of Swami Dayananda Krupa Home. He holds a Master of Science in Development Psychology and multiple certificates in Clinical Psychology, Applied Behaviour Analysis, Behaviour Modification, Sensory Integration, Feuerstein Remedial Methodology, and Special Education. He is a registered rehabilitation professional associated with the Rehab Council of India. Giridhar is based out of Chennai.

P. L. T. Girija
<sanjeevanifoundation@gmail.com>

Dr. P. L. T. Girija acquired her M.Phil. in Sociology from Jawaharlal Nehru University before pursuing a Bachelor of Ayurvedic Medicine and Surgery (BAMS) from Venkataramana Ayurveda College. This transition was inspired by her deep conviction that Ayurveda—an ancient medical system that has served Indian communities for millennia—offers safe, effective, and culturally rooted healthcare capable of addressing India's contemporary health challenges. Dr. Girija has built a distinguished career as an Ayurvedic physician, teacher, author, and public health advocate, combining rigorous academic grounding with decades of clinical experience and social commitment.

She is the founder of Sanjeevani Ayurveda and Yoga Centre and the Sanjeevani Foundation, institutions that have become important platforms for authentic Ayurvedic healthcare, clinical practice, and community outreach. Through these initiatives, she has consistently demonstrated how Ayurveda can provide accessible and affordable care while remaining rooted in its classical knowledge systems. She served as a consultant to the Health Systems Development Project of the Government of Tamil Nadu during 2004–2005 and also advised the Government on strategies for mainstreaming Ayurveda. She was instrumental in developing a state-level health kit integrating Ayurvedic and Siddha remedies, now distributed widely across Tamil Nadu. As part of her training initiatives, she helped train nearly 2,500 Village Health Nurses across the state in the principles and practical application of Ayurveda and Yoga, thereby strengthening grassroots healthcare delivery.

Widely recognised as one of the most prominent Ayurveda practitioners in Tamil Nadu, Dr. Girija has been invited to lecture and interact with students and scholars at several leading academic and research institutions across India. Her lectures have addressed both clinical practice and the broader role of Ayurveda in contemporary healthcare systems. Her clinical work was particularly notable during the first two waves of the COVID-19 pandemic, when she and her team treated more than one thousand COVID-19 patients, including individuals with multiple co-morbidities, using standalone Ayurvedic protocols. The outcomes were subsequently documented in peer-reviewed journals, contributing to the emerging evidence base on Ayurveda in pandemic response.

Her contributions have been recognised through several awards and honours. In 2009–2010, the Sanjeevani Ayurveda and Yoga Centre was recognised as a Centre of Excellence by the Department of AYUSH, Government of India. She received the Best Doctor Award in 2012 from Tamil Nadu Dr. M.G.R. Medical University and was honoured with the Bhishak Sri Award by Sri Sri College of Ayurvedic Science and Research, becoming the first woman Ayurveda practitioner to receive this recognition. In 2026, she was conferred the distinction of Fellow by the Rashtriya Ayurveda Vidyapeeth under the Ministry of AYUSH.

A prolific writer and communicator, Dr. Girija has authored numerous peer-reviewed research papers, medical articles, and opinion pieces in both national and regional publications. Her books include *Ayulai Valarkkum Ayurvedam* (Tamil, 2003), *Jeevani: Ayurveda for Women* (2013), and *Ayurveda for Revitalising Healthcare in India* (2017), reflecting her commitment to making Ayurvedic knowledge accessible to both practitioners and the wider public while advocating a more prominent role for Ayurveda within India's healthcare system.

Guriqbal Singh
<guriqbaldu@gmail.com>

Guriqbal Singh acquired his Bachelor's Degree in Sociology from Delhi University. He also holds a post-graduate diploma in Liberal Arts from Ashoka University. He heads Civic Action Lab, a social innovation and civic engagement initiative dedicated to co-creating solutions for community development, rural transformation, and participatory governance. The initiative undertakes applied and policy-oriented research, combining immersive field engagement with academic rigour to inform sustainable, inclusive development practices. Guriqbal is based out of New Delhi.

Dr Hardik S. Khamar
<drhardik@gmail.com>

Dr Hardik S. Khamar is a distinguished homeopathic physician, educator, and researcher, known for his expertise in chronic disease management, neurodevelopmental disorders, and integrative healthcare. With an MD in Homeopathy and certifications in Health & Family Welfare Management (New Delhi), Design Thinking (IIT Delhi), and SCMT (Germany), he combines traditional homeopathy with modern scientific advancements. As the Founder of Homeopathy Care Clinics, Ahmedabad, Dr Khamar specialises in treating cancers, autoimmune disorders, epilepsy, autism, ADHD, and lifestyle diseases. He is also a visiting faculty in Materia Medica at Sardar Patel University, a Board of Studies member at Swaminarayan University, and a panel doctor at the National Institute of Design, Ahmedabad. Dr Khamar has presented at prestigious international conferences, including the LMHI Congress (Turkey), the Ukrainian Homeopathic Congress, and the International Conference on Integrative Oncology (Kerala). He has delivered keynote addresses at Parul University, the AYUSH Department (Government of Gujarat), and the Ahmedabad Management Association, focusing on homeopathy's role in chronic disease, pseudo-surgical conditions, and Long COVID management. A reviewer for *Homeopathic Links* (Thieme Publishers) and a resource speaker for AYUSH, he actively contributes to research, faculty training, and policy discussions. His expertise in design thinking enables him to integrate homeopathy with Medicine 1.0 to 4.0, bridging traditional healing with modern healthcare advancements. Beyond medicine, Dr Khamar is an avid paraglider with over 270 hours of flying experience and an Ultimate Frisbee enthusiast. With his innovative approach and commitment to evidence-based homeopathy, he continues to shape the future of integrative medicine globally.

James Oliver
<j.oliver@rmit.edu.au>

James Oliver is a transdisciplinary educator and cultural collaborator with more than 20 years of research, teaching and engagement practice (including in the public sector across the arts and well-being). This has nurtured his research and creative practices, intersecting with community and cultural enquiry, and an advancement of 'practice as research' methodology. Another important aspect of James' work is in the area of Indigenous Practice Research, in international context and collaboration. This has developed from his formative understanding of place and land within his native community, culture, and language, and in the Scottish Hebrides. This cultural emplacement has also expanded through collaborations with practitioners and educators across Australia, Canada, Europe, India, and Japan. He is an Associate Professor in the School of Design, RMIT University, Melbourne.

Onkar Mittal

<o_mittal@rediffmail.com>

Dr Onkar Mittal is a social health activist with over four decades of experience. He worked at grassroots level for raising the voice of the poor to develop an understanding of social praxis with his colleagues and civil society. He also worked with government and donor-development agencies, including the UNICEF, WHO-India and DFID India, on a range of sectoral issues in urban basic services, health sector reform, RMNCH, water and sanitation, disaster prevention and relief, to name a few. He worked as a health advisor to DFID India from 1995 to 2003. He was with DFID-UK in London in 2001 when the MDG were being worked out. For the past two decades, he has been working independently on health policy and governance issues in Delhi, UP, Bihar, and Jharkhand. His current work on governance is focused around access to health, water, and river protection.

Purnima Arun
<purnimasarun@gmail.com>

Purnima Arun is a practitioner of simple and vernacular, season- appropriate, and traditional practices to ensure health and well-being. She learnt several recipes from her late husband, Shri Arun Kumar (Paani Baba), who was an expert in the traditional system of cooking desi food. Purnima has also spent several years learning about Ayurveda and connecting with health and food from late Dr S. D. Sharma, the deeply knowledgeable holistic healer who served tens of thousands of people who came to him for healing. Purnima offers a comprehensive course, "*Swad Aur Sehat*", on customised health and food regime for the individual in both online and physical retreat modes. Purnima is based out of Ghaziabad.

Rashmi Raut Gadgil
<rashmiraut3r@gmail.com>

Dr Rashmi Raut-Gadgil embarked on her medical journey after graduating from Government Medical

College, Nagpur, in 2008. Her early experiences included attending the Sevankur Youth Inspiration Camp and visiting various organisations and individuals working in tribal sectors, which instilled in her a deep sense of social responsibility and motivation to serve in rural India. She further explored this path through visits to trusts and hospitals focused on rural health and traditional medicine. Despite having the opportunity to pursue specialised MD/MS courses, Dr Raut-Gadgil chose to complete a Fellowship in Family Medicine at Christian Medical College, Vellore, from 2015 to 2017. This training equipped her to work effectively in resource-constrained settings, with expertise in Internal Medicine, Obstetrics-Gynaecology, Paediatrics, Emergency Care, and Preventive Care. Dr Raut-Gadgil has served as a medical officer in government rural hospitals and played a significant role as Nodal Officer at a tehsil-level Covid Care Centre, where her work was recognised by the district administration. During the pandemic, she also voluntarily treated critical Covid patients and worked at a semi-government Covid Care Centre, where she began to explore the integration of traditional medicine practices like Ayurveda with modern medicine. Currently, Dr Raut-Gadgil operates her own clinic in Ajara, Maharashtra, providing holistic treatment with a rational approach to various therapies. She is writing a book in Marathi on women's health. She is also expanding her knowledge by studying Ayurveda under Vaidyaraj Dr C. B. Desai.

Rhea D'Souza
<rhea@kabilaconsulting.com>

Rhea is an artist and the CEO of Kabila Consulting, an organisation and a movement committed to bridging the ecological, social, and spiritual divides, in order to contribute to building an interconnected world by design. As a naturalist and a polymath, she thrives in bringing different perspectives, especially from nature, to see more and allow emergence to happen. She is a believer of "Practice as an encounter" to see more. A doula, bridge, mother, wife, coach, sister, friend…she is based in Mumbai (as of now).

Riddhi Mehar
<riddhi.mehar@gmail.com>

A Doordarshan- graded and SPIC-MACAY- empanelled Kathak artist, Riddhi is a professionally trained Kathak dancer and educator, with over 22 years of experience in teaching and performing. A disciple of Guru Pt. Rajendra Gangani *ji*, she has also trained under eminent gurus and performed across India, with her practice rooted in the Gurukul Parampara and blended with contemporary, inclusive pedagogy. Founder of *Anaadikruti*, she also runs this Delhi-based classical arts initiative that promotes Indian dance as a tool for self-transformation, wellness, and cultural dialogue.

Ritu Priya Mehrotra
<ritupriyajnu@gmail.com>

Ritu Priya is a retired professor from the Centre of Social Medicine & Community Health, Jawaharlal Nehru University, New Delhi, India. A medical graduate with a Ph.D. in Community Health, her work links epidemiology, political economy, popular culture, and health systems research for decentralised planning, policy formulation and analysis. Her work has specifically focused on an eco-social epidemiological approach to urban health, health of marginalised groups, problems of nutrition, and communicable diseases. She also works on inter-disciplinary research methodologies, health technology assessment, and the ethics of public health. She was Advisor (Public Health Planning) with the National Health Systems Resource Centre, a technical support institution under the National Rural Health Mission, for two years and has been a member of task forces of the Planning Commission, the Department of Health and Family Welfare, the Ministry/Department of AYUSH, and the National AIDS Control Organisation in India. She is founding member of the Trans-disciplinary Research Cluster for Sustainability Studies and the Trans-disciplinary Research Cluster on Plural Health Care at Jawaharlal Nehru University.

Vijayaraghavan M. Chariar

<chariarv@iitd.ac.in>

Prof. Vijayaraghavan M. Chariar is a faculty member at the Indian Institute of Technology, Delhi. While Prof. Chariar's basic training is in experimental materials science, over the last two decades, he has worked on diverse areas such as Traditional Knowledge Systems, Design for Sustainability, Ecological Sanitation, Appropriate Housing, and Joyous Leadership. Prof. Chariar uses an experiential and learner-centred approach in his pedagogy and has inspired a large number of students to achieve their highest innate potential, several of whom have taken to entrepreneurship in the social sector. For his innovative pedagogy, Prof. Chariar was awarded the Teaching Excellence Award by IIT Delhi in 2011. Prof. Chariar taught and researched at Arizona State University as a Fulbrighter in 2012-2013. In addition to IIT Delhi, he is much loved by students at BITS Pilani, IIT Kharagpur, and School of Planning & Architecture, New Delhi. He is the author of several patents, publications, technical manuals, and design registrations on innovative technologies. Prof. Chariar serves as Chairman of IIT Delhi's much awarded sanitation start-up, Ekam Eco Solutions, and also mentors several startups. Prof. Chariar lovingly creates impact in water, sanitation, and well-being through IITD-partnered ventures Ekam Eco Solutions and JoyIsYou. He has been a sought-after invited speaker by diverse academic, volunteering, and corporate institutions on topics including sustainability, start-ups, and self- discovery. At IIT Delhi, he teaches various courses, including Design Thinking & Innovation, Rural Innovation & Entrepreneurship, Traditional Knowledge & Values, and Technology Alternatives for Rural Development. In his research group, Frugal Innovation JoyLab, research scholars from diverse disciplines work closely with communities of farmers, artisans, and forest dwellers to collaboratively develop culturally acceptable and time-tested innovative solutions with a focus on community adoption and translation.